EDUCATING MEDICAL TEACHERS

This volume is published as part of a long-standing cooperative program between the Harvard University Press and the Commonwealth Fund, a philanthropic foundation, to encourage the publication of significant scholarly books in medicine and health.

Educating Medical Teachers

GEORGE E. MILLER, M.D.

 A COMMONWEALTH FUND BOOK

HARVARD UNIVERSITY PRESS
CAMBRIDGE, MASSACHUSETTS
AND LONDON, ENGLAND
1980

Library of Congress Cataloging in Publication Data

Miller, George E
    Educating medical teachers.

    "A Commonwealth Fund book."
    Includes index.
    1.   Medical education—Teacher training.   I.   Title.
R833.5.M53   610'.7   79-26148
ISBN 0-674-23775-7

To three valued mentors

Granville A. Bennett
Ward Darley
Lester J. Evans

ACKNOWLEDGMENTS

This book was undertaken at the persistent urging of colleagues who seemed to feel that the evolution of educational research, development, and teacher training efforts in medicine was a story that should be told before my memory and my files fell victim to the inevitable deterioration that accompanies the lengthening years. Chief among them was Tamas Fulop, director of the Division of Health Manpower Development at the World Health Organization in Geneva. William J. Grove, now vice chancellor for academic affairs at the University of Illinois at the Medical Center, a close collaborator for twenty years in his successive roles as a faculty member, associate dean, dean, and executive dean of the College of Medicine, provided the encouragement and the freedom that made the task of writing seem possible. Phillip M. Forman, my successor as director of the Center for Educational Development, eased the transition back into academic pursuits and by his support made this work much easier.

Many others contributed both conceptually and substantively as the writing progressed. Among those to whom I am particularly grateful for reviewing portions of the book that touched upon their contributions are Stephen Abrahamson, Granville Bennett, Edward Bridge, Julius Comroe, Cecilia Conrath (Doak), Ward Darley, Lester Evans, Jose Ferreira, Reginald Fitz, Hilliard Jason, Fred Katz, Edwin Rosinski, and Paul Sanazaro. It was helpful to have their comments and suggestions, but none of them need feel any responsibility for the interpretative reporting of events in which they were involved; that burden is mine alone.

Among those who contributed in other ways I must give special thanks to Robert Chrismer, whose skill in seeking out original documents made the assembly of background materials seem so simple; to Martha Urban, whose editorial suggestions were so helpful; and to Greer Williams, whose observations and advice from the view of a professional writer were so illuminating. Maria Pintado, Roxanne Engel, and Dawn Lippeth also deserve special acknowledgment for their patient and faithful typing and retyping of draft after draft of the manuscript. It is also fitting to express my appreciation to the Carnegie Foundation for the Advancement of Teaching and to the World Health Organization for permission to quote extensively from copyrighted works.

The Commonwealth Fund supported so many pieces of the work described here that it might better be thought of as a partner than as merely a benefactor. I am grateful not only for that long-term interest but also for the most recent grant-in-aid to assist in the preparation of this book, which aims to bring it all together. The Rockefeller Foundation has also won warm thanks for providing me with a month-long retreat as a scholar-in-residence at the Villa Serbelloni, where the book was at last completed.

And finally, 1 am grateful to my wife for her patience over the years while the work was being done; her understanding while the task of writing was under way; and her critical suggestions at important moments before some unpardonable gaffe was committed.

G.E.M.

CONTENTS

EDUCATING MEDICAL TEACHERS

INTRODUCTION

The question of the preparation of college teachers is a
high explosive. Toss it into any academic gathering and
the air is instantly filled with the shattered fragments of
human dignity, and with cries of triumph and despair.

—*Samuel P. Capen (1938)*

A wiser man might have heeded Chancellor Capen's warning and
sought a less hazardous occupation than educating medical teachers
(some might add, a more useful one as well). But hazard and utility
aside, there seemed little question at the start that it was worthwhile
work; twenty-five years later the conviction is undiminished. This
account of what happened during that interval may lead others to
the same conclusion.

It is curious that so many of our most important responsibilities are undertaken without significant preparation. Marriage and
parenthood are probably the most ubiquitous illustrations, and
there is little reason to expect that these states, based as they are on
the elusive chemistry of emotion, will ever evolve rationally. The
task of medical teaching, on the other hand, is accepted deliberately
and dispassionately, yet the preparation for that influential role is
equally frail. Such an opinion, however, is where the combat begins.

As a young internist climbing the conventional academic ladder,
using a research laboratory and a metabolic unit as important rungs
to support the ascent, I realized only slowly that in the accompanying function of teacher I was behaving very much like my own medical school teachers — and it was not clear whether either they or I
fully understood what we were about. Despite a genuine interest in
helping students to become physicians, it is a tradition among faculty members to assume that a sound personal base in biomedical science and clinical medicine is adequate preparation for that work.
The assignment is further complicated by the fact that most stu-

dents are aiming for a professional life of medical practice very different from that chosen by their most influential mentors. The high level of anxiety experienced by so many medical students in the course of this study is not unfamiliar to the teaching staff, many of whom are inclined to view the feeling as an inevitable part of the educational system, one that at least the medically qualified among them successfully weathered and thus an experiencing that is almost certainly good for those they teach. The epithets like "rat race" that students use in describing the curriculum, or the frequency with which they appear to regard the early years more as a sentence than an opportunity, produce tolerant sounds of sympathy and even some fine tuning of program organization and instructional methods. Not until the Western Reserve revolution, however, was timidity replaced by audacity as more and more medical schools took up the search for a better arrangement of course content and sequence. The number of man-years that have gone into curriculum manipulation during the last two decades is surely staggering. And the disappointment that too often followed must be far greater than has been generally acknowledged, even though the evidence of reversion to earlier patterns is all around us.

Healthy as such efforts were, potentially useful as they may have been, it is increasingly clear that the design and implementation of many new instructional programs resembles nothing so much as building a new home and then living the same old life within it. The architecture may be admirable, but the social interactions are often deplorable. If that aspect of education is to be altered then the actors, not merely the stage setting, probably need attention as well.

So goes the argument for educating medical teachers as teachers, not as biomedical scientists or medical practitioners alone. That work is what this book is about. It is not intended as a manual for pedagogues in medicine but as an account of how the concept evolved, the problems that were encountered, the alternatives that demanded consideration, and the challenges that still remain. Along the way some of the traditional values that medical academicians hold dear have had to be questioned. Among the most important are those which underlie a growing conflict between the academic and social purposes of medical schools and medical schooling. The questions are painful, but inescapable; the answers are often equally so.

There are those who have looked disdainfully upon this educational research and development effort as a passing fad, a semireligious movement whose fervor would peak and pass. And certainly there have been those among us who exhibited an almost missionary need to convert the nonbelievers. Most, however, have recognized in the discipline of education a new set of tools with which to probe old and still perplexing problems of medical education, as well as new ones. And the function of tools, in contrast to weapons, is not to win battles but to facilitate the achievement of more constructive goals. The new breed of medical educationist, accepting such a supporting role which has to be played more in the wings than in the spotlight, soon learns that one of the most difficult parts of the job is being patient. Even after more than a score of years on the front line, impatience is among my most implacable enemies.

This feeling may show through here and there, for in spite of an unremitting effort to make this interpretative history objective, and nonjudgmental, it is also very personal. As such, the narrative is subject to all the distortion of that unique lens through which an involved author sees things. Because it is written in the first person, it may also suggest a greater personal claim for credit than is either contemplated or justified. I can do no more than acknowledge the possibility, while denying the intent.

What I cannot deny is the still provocative nature of much that is captured here. Education is still a soft science in the eyes of many hard-headed medical teachers, one that must prove its worth before being admitted as an equal into the walled world of medicine. Yet those who are most insistent in this demand seem least likely to accept as "proof" any evidence that is not gathered through the conventional hypothesis-testing experimental model in which one variable at a time is manipulated. Unfortunately, medical education is rarely susceptible to that kind of artificial study. And when a tiny piece is teased out for such meticulous examination, the results are commonly dismissed because they fail to take into consideration what occurs in the real world. The medical educationist who tries to defend what is indefensible soon loses credibility as well as the argument; the one who succumbs to conventional wisdom about research will end studying controllable things of academic elegance but of practical insignificance. It is wiser to acknowledge — nay, to insist — that the experimental model is generally unsuited to this task, without apologizing for systematic studies of equal rigor that are descriptive or analytic in nature. For these, too, produce a data base, one that is far more secure than the opinions and preferences and traditions that underlie so much that is now prescribed in the name of medical education, and defended in the name of "quality," without a shred of evidence beyond the firm beliefs of distinguished academicians who *know* what is right, even if they are unable to prove it.

Shifting such attitudes of personal certainty about educational process toward individual and institutional attitudes of inquiry is the goal of educating medical teachers. The work is not designed to spread a new orthodoxy about curriculum or instruction or evaluation but to foster doubt, to facilitate discovery, and to nourish change. Perhaps this account of how it evolved in the last quarter century will bring a perspective that is useful in planning for the next. At least that is my hope.

IDEAS WITHOUT ACTION

1

The origin of an idea, a technique, a movement, is often difficult to discern. If they were pressed to describe where it all began, many contemporary workers in the field of research in medical education might agree with Ward Darley, late executive director of the Association of American Medical Colleges, who wrote: "The first organized effort to study and evaluate the broad spectrum of the teaching and learning processes in medicine was developed as the Project in Medical Education at the University of Buffalo in 1955."[1] Certainly those who took part in that heady experience often felt like pioneers, even though they were sometimes described in far less flattering terms.

But the simple truth is that what occurred in a small, provincial university represented at most the flowering of an idea whose time had come. The seed, planted long before, had been nurtured by many individuals, in many places, who were somehow unable to generate or sustain the forces that would have made it grow and thrive. At Buffalo the combination of people and circumstances proved to be right, but without the rising tide of interest in the process of medical teaching and learning that had been generated by others, this fertile mixture might never have taken root. To understand how it came about requires a look into the past — a past generously sprinkled with ideas but lacking any sustained action.

It would be hard to say who first called attention to the distinction between what is taught in medical schools and how it is taught (or learned). In modern times the distinguished German surgeon Theo-

dor Billroth was surely among the leaders. His 1876 book on medical education, *Lehren und Lernen der Medicinishen Wissenschaft-
en* ("Teaching and Learning of Medical Knowledge"),[2] even anticipated the title of a now standard reference work that emerged
seventy-five years later from the Buffalo experience. In his account
of middle European and particularly of German medical education,
Billroth noted that as early as 1811 the Austrian Imperial Commission on Schools had issued "An Order for the Establishment of
Training Schools for Future Professors of Medicine and Related Sciences." In practice, these institutes appeared to focus on ensuring in
their graduates the highest level of achievement in the sciences, with
scant attention paid to the means by which these teachers would
then instruct their own students. It was this emphasis that may have
led Billroth to point out that "in teaching, and especially in teaching large groups, the importantce of form and method must not be
underestimated. On the contrary, we must acknowledge their great
pedagogical significance, and therefore spare no effort to perfect
them."[3] But the ensuing literature gives no hint that anything was
done to translate Billroth's apparent concern for pedagogy into educational practices in Germanic institutions of the time.

Similar concerns were brewing in the New World, particularly in
Chicago and Boston. E. L. Holmes, addressing the 1892 annual
banquet of the Practitioners Club in Chicago, was reported to say:
"Despite the great advances in American medical education during
the last few years, it still remains a painful fact that the methods of
teaching in our colleges are unphilosophical and the means of instruction lamentably inadequate. A trade can scarcely be mentioned in which young men are taught their work in so irregular a
manner as they are taught the theory and practice of medicine."
Unfortunately, the solution he suggested would scarcely match the
best in pedagogy that was known even then: "What is needed to improve the instruction in our medical schools is . . . the addition to
the usual corps of professors [of] a large number of instructors similar in function to drill masters in the army."[4]

In the same year an editorial in the *Journal of the American Medical Association* noted a general discomfort among medical educators, stating: "It is quite evident that there is a feeling of unrest and
anxiety for better methods of teaching medicine on the part of the
most experienced teachers."[5]

This discomfort apparently produced no significant effect, for seven years later Dr. Bayard Holmes, professor of surgery at the University of Illinois College of Physicians and Surgeons, wrote:

Teachers of medicine have been paying too much attention to the subjects and too little to the students they are teaching and to the manner in which they are doing it . . . The medical student, after years of cramming and dissecting, section making and hunting unknowns, finds himself utterly unable to cope with the simplest problems of diagnosis and treatment. This state of affairs has caused many teachers to look back with longing to the old days of the preceptor and the short course of medical lectures, but it has led others to bestir themselves and study the pedagogic problems which have been working themselves out for a long time in other departments of education.[6]

Even medical students began to take up the cry. The observations made by one of them are particularly significant, since Walter B. Cannon later became one of America's most distinguished medical scientists. In 1900, however, he wrote from the vantage point that student status provides: "Among many instructors there is manifest dissatisfaction with the traditional means of training physicians, a dissatisfaction rising apparently from the belief that the teaching of medicine has not been keeping pace with improvements in the teaching of other subjects. Discussion of old methods and earnest searching after new and more effective methods of preparing young men to be practitioners are consequently rife amongst us."[7]

Cannon's voice was not alone at Harvard. The eminent internist Richard C. Cabot noted in a 1905 issue of the *Boston Medical and Surgical Journal* that "given good teachers and abundant material for teaching, the benefits acquired by the student can be enormously increased by good methods of instruction or diminished by poor ones." Two of the specific suggestions Cabot made for improving medical instruction have the sound of contemporary wisdom. Referring to the evaluation of teaching he wrote:

Medical teaching like most university teaching is greatly in need of supervision and criticism. All teaching up to and through the high school is properly visited, supervised and criticised. In collegiate and postgraduate work there is in most universities no adequate system of supervision, and medical schools have to bear their part in this great evil. Should an intelligent visitor come to the Harvard Medical School, study the methods of teaching medicine and visit the classes systematically for a

week or two, he would know more of what was being done, well
or ill, than any living man knows today. Today no one's work
is inspected, praised or corrected. Only by inquiring of students
is any idea gained of what the teachers are doing, whether they
do it well or ill, and whether their courses duplicate or overlap.

In reference to examinations, he pointed out:

Examinations should be a practical test of the students' power
to diagnose and treat disease, in short to practice medicine, not
his power to write or talk about medicine. Some men who have
never learned the art of writing examinations make the best
practitioners. The powers of such men would be shown in their
true light if the examination consisted of the examination,
diagnosis and treatment of cases. On the other hand those glib
students who can write and talk fluently about disease but cannot hear, see or feel the signs of disease, nor sensibly advise a
patient, would also be fairly tested as at present they are not.

The highest purpose of the examination is, we believe, to indicate to him who has in charge the instruction of the student,
his acquirements and needs.[8]

But perhaps most significant was the interest evidenced by the Association of American Medical Colleges (AAMC). In 1901 the president of that association said at the annual meeting: "It seems to me
as I get the perspective of the work of our Association more in view,
that in the future it will be along educational lines. We must introduce better methods of teaching; we must study medical pedagogy.
Our work should be a helpful, inspiring and educational one, rather
than a political one. Our session should be in the nature of postgraduate work in teaching teachers how to teach. We should have
more educational and pedagogic sessions."[9] This further observation appeared in the proceedings of the annual meeting for 1904:
"There probably never was a time when methods of teaching were so
important as now. In arts and sciences other than medicine they are
undergoing most careful scrutiny, development and reconstruction.
They are being considered from psychologic, pedagogic, and practical aspects. Every effort is being made to determine how to con-
serve energy and to secure the best results with the means at hand
and for the purpose in view."[10]

By 1908 interest in these questions had apparently grown to such
a point that a standing AAMC Committee on Medical Teaching was
appointed. It was specifically charged with "consideration of the

pedagogic elements in medical education, with special reference to the training of medical teachers, methods of instruction employed, and allied topics." These noble words were apparently followed by limited deeds, however, for there is little in the AAMC archives to suggest that the committee engaged in any significant action.

The year 1910 is generally regarded as a landmark in medical education, for it was then that the Carnegie Foundation for the Advancement of Teaching published *Bulletin Number Four: Medical Education in the United States and Canada*. Abraham Flexner's savage attack, thoroughly documented and skillfully presented, did far more than destroy whatever illusions might have existed about the quality of medical schools and medical schooling; it also recommended program revisions that have served as a reference point for medical educators for more than fifty years. Although the document is strangely silent on the means of preparing faculty members to implement the instructional practices Flexner envisioned, the vision itself provides ample guidelines for such training. For example, in describing the opportunities that must be given to students in academic programs, he said:

> On the pedagogic side, modern medicine, like all scientific teaching, is characterized by activity. The student no longer merely watches, listens, memorizes; he does. His own activities in the laboratory and in the clinic are the main factors in his instruction and discipline. An education in medicine nowadays involves both learning and learning how; the student cannot effectively know unless he knows how.[11]

Flexner was equally direct in commenting on teachers and their responsibilities:

> From the standpoint of the young student, the school is, of course, concerned chiefly with his acquisition of the proper knowledge, attitude, and technique. Once more, it matters not at that stage whether his destination is to be investigation or practice. In either case, as beginner, he learns chiefly what is old, known, understood. But the old, known, and understood are all alike new to him; and the teacher in presenting it to his apprehension seeks to evoke the attitude, and to carry him through the processes, of the thinker and not of the parrot.
> The student is throughout to be kept on his mettle. He does not have to be a passive learner, just because it is too early for

him to be an original explorer. He can actively master and se-
curely fix scientific technique and method in the process of ac-
quiring the already known. From time to time a novel turn may
indeed give zest to routine; but the undergraduate student of
medicine will for the most part acquire the methods, standards,
and habits of science by working over territory which has been
traversed before, in an atmosphere freshened by the search for
truth.[12]

This reference to the search for truth as a characteristic of any
university, of which medical schools must be a part, is a consistent
thread throughout the fabric of this report. Thus Flexner insists
upon the critical importance of a research spirit among faculty
members, whatever the setting for their principal work may be:

Teachers of modern medicine, clinical as well as scientific,
must then be men of active, progressive temper, with definite
ideals, exacting habits in thought and work, and with still some
margin for growth. No considerable part of their energy and
time is indeed absorbed in what is after all routine instruction;
for their situation differs vastly from that of workers in non-
teaching institutions devoted wholly to investigation. Their
practical success depends, therefore, on their ability to carry
into routine the rigor and the vigor of their research moments.
A happy adjustment is in this matter by no means easy; nor has
it been as yet invariably reached. Investigators, impressed with
the practical importance of scientific method to the practising
physician, tend perhaps to believe that it is to be acquired only
in original research. A certain impatience therefore develops,
and ill-equipped student barks venture prematurely into un-
charted seas. But the truth is that an instructor, devoting part
of his day under adequate protection to investigation, can
teach even the elements of his subject on rigorously scientific
lines.[13]

However, Flexner is far more careful than some of his followers to
maintain a sense of balance about the qualities to be sought in
teachers and the purposes to be served by a medical school:

On the other hand, it will never happen that every professor in
either the medical school or the university faculty is a genuinely
productive scientist. There is room for men of another type—

the non-productive assimilative teacher of wide learning, continuous receptivity, critical sense, and responsive interest. Not
infrequently these men, catholic in their sympathies, scholarly
in spirit and method, prove the purveyors and distributors
through whom new ideas are harmonized and made current.
They preserve balance and make connections.[14]

Flexner was also careful to remind his readers that "the business
of the medical school is the making of doctors; nine-tenths of its
graduates will . . . never be anything else." Thus he both anticipated and tried to deal realistically with the battle that has continued to this day about the relative importance of basic and applied
sciences in medical education:

Anatomy and physiology are ultimately biological sciences. Do
the professional purposes of the medical school modify the
strict biological point of view? Should the teaching of anatomy
and physiology be affected by the fact that these subjects are
parts of a medical curriculum? Or ought they be presented
exactly as they would be presented to students of biology not in-
tending to be physicians? A layman hesitates to offer an opinion
where the doctors disagree, but the purely pedagogical standpoint may assist a determination of the issue. Perhaps a certain
misconception of what is actually at stake is in a measure responsible for the issue. Scientific rigor and thoroughness are
not in question. Whatever the point of view — whether purely
biological or medical — scientific method is equally feasible and
essential; a verdict favorable to recognition of the explicitly
medical standpoint would not derogate from scientific rigor.
    . . . research, untrammeled by near reference to practical
ends, will go on in every properly organized medical school; its
critical method will dominate all teaching whatsoever; but
undergraduate instruction will be throughout explicitly con-
scious of its professional end and aim. In no other way can all
the sciences belonging to the medical curriculum be thoroughly
kneaded. An active apperceptive relation must be established
and maintained between laboratory and clinical experience.
Such a relation cannot be one-sided; it will not spontaneously
set itself up in the last two years if it is deliberately suppressed in
the first two. There is no cement like interest, no stimulus like
the hint of a coming practical application.[15]

And finally, he pointed out to teachers and learners alike:

> In methods of instruction there is, once more, nothing to distinguish medical from other sciences. Out-and-out didactic treatment is hopelessly antiquated; it belongs to an age of accepted dogma or supposedly complete information, when the professor "knew" and the students "learned." The lecture indeed continues of limited use.[16]

Profound changes in medical education occurred in the decade following the Flexner report, but they were chiefly changes in institutional setting, curriculum organization, subject matter content, and faculty credentials. The pedagogic message that ran through so mcuh of the report was either overlooked or ignored. It was only an occasional medical faculty member, caught up in this new wave of scientifically based medical education, who paused to reflect on the process of instruction. One of these was E. P. Lyon, dean and professor of physiology at the University of Minnesota School of Medicine, who wrote in 1916:

> I try to believe that our poor results are due to poor training in the premedical years, or in high school or earlier still. I try to convince myself of the inherited inability of many to observe or think logically. I try to persuade myself that we turn over to the clinical teachers a pretty good product, and that the latter destroy our work by methods of didacticism, empiricism and worship of authority. Nevertheless, with all due allowance I come back to the physiology laboratory in fear and humility, for I feel that better pedagogic leadership would give better results. I wonder whether we shall some day have medical normal schools and teachers who shall teach us how to teach.[17]

Lyon's concern for this aspect of medical attention must have become generally known, because by 1923 his name was included among the members of a newly labeled AAMC Committee on Education and Pedagogics. Although there is virtually nothing in the literature to suggest that this committee had any significant impact on national educational practices, Dean Lyon's personal influence was surely being felt at home. For a brief period during the late 1920s, the University of Minnesota must have been going through much the same kind of introspective ferment that occurred at the Unversity of Buffalo thirty years later. For what appears to have been the first time, a sustained dialogue between the faculties of medicine and education was established at Minnesota. But the communication was more than talk; it represented joint work on a common problem, that of improving medical instruction. The first result was reported in the January 1929 *Journal of the Association of American Medical Colleges*. Significantly, one of the two papers was written by the dean of the College of Education, the second by a professor of pharmacology in the School of Medicine.

To those who regarded professional educators as starry-eyed or muddle-headed, it must have come as a great surprise to have Dean M. E. Haggerty report the results of an educational experiment in medicine, and to "plead for research in teaching problems . . . as a supplement to that body of knowledge which individual experience has so fruitfully contributed." Haggerty then went on to present the results of controlled experiments set up to determine the benefit of the laboratory experience in physiology and anatomy that had for so long been supported solely by the "individual experience" of a teaching faculty. Although the data did not support the faculty's faith in that instructional method, there is nothing to suggest that either curriculum structure or faculty behavior at Minnesota was altered by the findings.

Dean Haggerty had introduced his report by saying: "More and more as one studies the problems of higher education it becomes increasingly clear that the solution of our teaching problems must be a joint enterprise of men trained in the techniques of educational research and of other men who are scholars in the fields of academic and practical knowledge." He concluded with these words: "If this proposal is taken seriously and prosecuted through a period of years, attacking problem after problem in the analytic and detailed fashion necessitated by the requirements of scientific method, then we may, in time, give definite and objective validation to many of our teaching procedures which as yet rest upon the warrant of personal experiences and individual judgement. In the process some of our most stoutly defended opinions will doubtless be worn away as illusions, but in the end our teaching practices will be improved and ennobled and will become the fit compeers of the scientific techniques in the practice of [medicine] itself."[18]

Even now it is refreshing to note that the plea for research came from a dean (and a dean of education at that), while the plea for practical application of established principles of learning came from a basic scientist. For Professor A. D. Hirschfelder's paper began by pointing out:

Today's medical student has had a thorough course in general chemistry, organic chemistry, and physical chemistry. He has performed the fundamental experiments with his own hands. He has done the same in the laboratory of physiological chemistry and of physiology. The theoretical aspects have been well covered in lectures, quizzes, and examinations. But he has usually taken these subjects as the necessary evils of a long curriculum, and by the time he enters his clinical years, they have been shed from his cortex like water off a duck's back. He has not learned to correlate them with the facts of the bedside because his teachers of chemistry and physiology have not intimated their practical usefulness, and it is only rarely that his clinical instructors have revived them with a definiteness sufficient to bring back the hazy recollections of his early training.

I would like to bring before you some of the methods which I have used at the University of Minnesota to bring about this result, and which I have found by experience actually do so to a considerable degree.[19]

Hirshfelder went on to describe a set of learning experiences that captured in practice such techniques for facilitating learning as the provision of advance organizers, discovery methods, self-assessment procedures, immediate feedback, and significant opportunity for transfer. He was wise enough to avoid the use of these technical terms in describing what he was up to, but they were unmistakably present in his program plans.

Although Minnesota clearly put into action a set of advanced ideas drawn from the science of education, that action must have come to an end shortly after these reports were published. There is no evidence in the medical education literature of continuity, nor is there any recollection of these events in the contemporary university memory system. It was a noble effort — advanced in concept, solid in principle — but for reasons lost in institutional history it did not survive.

The general pace of interest in these ideas did quicken, however, during the decade of the thirties, and the quickening must have reflected, in some part at least, the impact of leaders such as Lyon, Hirschfelder, and Haggerty. Irving S. Cutter, dean of the Medical School at Northwestern University, was particularly blunt in calling attention to the need for improvement in teaching practices, saying that "of a given faculty possibly 5% have natural teaching ability. A larger percentage may, however, become excellent teachers through the application of a few elementary principles of pedagogy."[20]

In another school, Russell Oppenheimer, dean of medicine at Emory University, pointed out the importance of keeping before members of a medical faculty the subject of the art of teaching, and learning from those in the Department of Pedagogy.[21] Even a national Commission on Medical Education, in a final report published in 1932, stated firmly that "The commission has believed from the beginning that an emphasis on educational principles in medical training and licensure can be secured only by modifying the point of view and broadening the interests of those responsible . . . not by recommendations, statistics, new regulations, legislation or manipulation of the curriculum . . . At the present time it is probably true that the ability to teach is not sufficiently considered in the selection of personnel of some faculties, and little attention is paid to the preparation of medical teachers in the art of teaching."[22]

But the most visionary event of the decade was probably a 1933 publication entitled *Teaching Methods in Medicine: The Application of the Philosphy of Contemporary Education to Medical School.* William D. Reid, the author of this unusual volume, was an assistant professor of cardiology at the Boston University School of Medicine. He must have possessed more than an average endowment of humility, for in reviewing his own performance as a teacher he said somewhat wistfully: "I thought favorably of my lectures to the third-year students until I observed their meager results when I taught the same individuals as seniors in the wards."[23]

In an earlier paper on the medical teacher, Reid had pointed out that "familiarity with the science of pedagogy is just as important to medical teachers as [to] those engaged in nonmedical education . . . The present need of medical faculties is not for more 'authorities' on medicine, but for more 'teachers.' We should be concerned not only with what we teach but how we teach it."[24]

Reid's personal search for a solution to this problem led to his enrollment in a course entitled Methods of Teaching and Curriculum Formation given by Professor Guy Wilson at the Boston University School of Education. It was apparently Wilson's inspiration and model that led Reid to write the book that a reviewer for the *Journal of the Association of American Medical Colleges* described in this way: "It is well known that nothing by way of a text on teaching medical subjects has been available . . . It is gratifying to know that someone has had the courage to tackle so fearsome a subject."[25]

The book was a straightforward and lucid discussion that dealt at length with such topics as the psychology of learning, conditions that affect learning, and major techniques of teaching, and summarized in language remarkably free of jargon the principal findings extracted from the science of education that had applicability in a medical school setting. But Reid was apparently a quarter century too early. There is no evidence that his book had an impact on medical education in general; even at his own school the work was apparently ignored. Senior faculty members who still remember Dr. Reid describe him as a scholarly man, but they are unable to recall that any of his ideas produced significant program changes. Certainly there is no indication in the Boston University archives that his book or his views were influential in curriculum development or modification of instructional practices. In fact his work was so little known that twenty-five years later the Buffalo group was unaware that it was replicating much of what Reid had already proposed.

During the 1940s and 1950s a notable surge of interest in the appraisal and improvement of medical teaching took place. Individuals, professional associations, national and international conferences and commissions called attention with increasing frequency to deficiencies in the pedagogical qualifications of medical teachers. More and more often, professional educators were given space in medical journals and air time at medical meetings to describe and document their expertise.

Perhaps even more than in the United States, faculty leaders in the United Kingdom exhibited concern for the problem. Such distinguished figures as the Regius Professor of Medicine at the University of Aberdeen, for example, cried out: "Teaching is an art and it would be strangely unique among the arts if it were not possible by study of its technique to better its performance."[26] The most vigorous British proponent of a more aggressive attack on the apparent deficiencies in medical teaching was R. D. Lawrence, a senior physician at King's College Hospital Medical School in London. In "The Training of Clinical Teachers," a paper presented to the Fellows of the Royal College of Physicians and later published in the *British Medical Journal,* Lawrence outlined the problem and a suggested solution in these words:

There is wide agreement that clinical medicine is supremely hard to teach, that the teachers are not trained, and that conquently their efficiency and their students suffer. I suggest that the following steps should be taken.

A special course on medical teaching must be established by concerted effort . . . In the first place the course would be short —perhaps a half-day for four weeks would suffice. It would be experimental—extremely so. If, in the first place, it only managed to improve the teachers' elocution and delivery it would have done enough to justify its existence. If it managed to inculcate general principles and an awareness of mental processes it would be doubly justified. In the long run I would hope that these teachers, getting together to form some group might evolve a philosophy of medical teaching and thought, produce a stimulating book on the subject, tackle the problem of the medical curriculum and promote the essential rewriting of text books. The whole medical world would be stimulated and benfitted.[27]

On the other side of the Atlantic, academic leaders such as Lawrence Slobody, professor of pediatrics at New York Medical College, and Russell Meyers, professor of surgery at the State University of Iowa, were sounding similar tocsins. In Slobody's view:

1. Effective medical teaching has not been developed to its fullest extent.
2. The principles of education have the same relationship to medical teaching as basic sciences have to clinical medicine.
3. The proper application of the principles of education will improve medical teaching.
4. Medical colleges should make the basic principles of education an integral part of the curriculum. A graduate course leading to a master's degree in medical education should be available to prospective teachers.[28]

Meanwhile Meyers, in a thoughtful and thoroughly documented review of educational science in medical teaching, came to the following conclusion:

In broad terms, the influence of educational science on medical teaching in the United States may be summarized by quoting briefly from pertinent articles of relatively recent date:

"We have advanced rapidly in all phases of medicine but slowly in medical teaching. It is time to improve our medical teaching by applying scientifically proved education principles based on careful research.

". . . in the professional schools, the teaching staffs and the curriculum committees . . . consist in large part of technically qualified experts whose interest in and familiarity with the science of education is lamentably small."

That this state of affairs prevails in the year 1953 may come as something of a surprise to the student of general education. Particularly if he supposes *a priori* that the chief function of a teacher in a college of medicine must be that of teaching and that medical teachers must surely have acquired the general background of pedagogic theory and communication skills available in the warehouse of educational science. Such supposition is, unfortunately, not rooted in fact. To be sure, exceptional individuals can be found who feel it incumbent to acquaint themselves with the field of general education as well as with their special areas of interest in the basic medical and clinical sciences. They are, however, almost unbelievably small in number.[29]

The professional educators were also cautiously inserting their views. A professor of education at the University of Leeds noted in the *British Medical Journal* that "as time goes on the need is likely to become more apparent for a closer linkage between institutes of education and the departments of medical schools."[30] Paul Klapper, writing in the *Journal of the Association of American Medical Colleges,* observed: "While the medical sciences have been rich and inviting fields for experimentation and research, medical education is still virgin terrain waiting for equally meticulous inquiry into the art of effective teaching of its materials."[31]

Even the medical education establishment began to voice such concern in its official conferences and publications. The final report of the Committee on Survey of Medical Education (which was established by the Association of American Medical Colleges and the American Medical Association) declared:

> Many of [the] forces and opinions influencing the curriculum have laid more emphasis on the facts to be taught . . . than on the guidance of the student in his learning process . . . The greatest need of the medical schools today is clear, critical thought by men who are sincerely interested in the education of students and who have an understanding of educational principles.[32]

And the medical curriculum committee of the British Medical Association noted in a formal document:

> The Committee would draw attention to a notable ommission in the training of the medical teacher. Although the science and practice of education have made great progress in recent years, and it is considered essential for most teachers in schools and colleges to have had special instruction and experience in the art of pedagogy, teachers in universities and medical schools receive no such training. Few are born teachers; most would benefit from such a course. Efforts should be made to remedy this defect by providing suitable courses in association with university departments of education.[33]

But the arguments were not all on this side. In a report of the First Teaching Institute of the Association of American Medical Colleges, Abraham White reflects the ambivalence of basic medical scientists about the question of providing special training in the art and science of education for future medical faculty members.[34] Having expressed forcefully the primary importance of assuring solid grounding in subject matter, the participants acknowledged that professional educators might be of some limited usefulness in improving instruction but that the greatest benefit would be derived from senior faculty members observing, critically evaluating, and providing constructive suggestions on the teaching done by their juniors. They were uniformly skeptical of the value of formal courses in pedagogy.

This skepticism was even expressed by some who later became strong supporters. For example, Ward Darley and Edward Turner said in 1949:

> It is safe to state that with few exceptions the teachers currently active in medical education have definitely not been developed as a result of any deliberate or formal preparation in the field of education.
>
> It is generally agreed that there are a few general principles which might be called pedagogical that can be applied in the medical program. It is logical, however, that medical faculties are distrustful of principles that have been arrived at by teaching young children or by studying rats and other laboratory animals.[35]

At the first World Conference on Medical Education, Professor W. Melville Arnott of the University of Birmingham Faculty of Medicine said with force and conviction:

A recurring complaint is that medical teachers are commonly chosen without much, if any, attention being paid to their pedagogic qualities. It is even suggested that these should be valued above all other attributes. While pedagogic facility is certainly an advantage, I maintain that it is a quite subsidiary qualification and not even essential in education at the University level. Far more important qualities in the University level teacher are intellectual honesty, discipline, curiosity, and love of scholarship. Without these, pedagogic ability becomes a grave handicap as it may so easily lead to the perversion of the young.[36]

In his presidential address to the Conference, Sir Lionel Whitby said with equal forcefulness: "Talents will be wasted or misused if the structure and content of medical education are faulty and if medical educationalists remain complacently satisfied with themselves and their methods."[37]

Thus the ferment evolved, with increasing words, an occasional piece of action, but never with the critical concentration of persuasive ideas and persuaded individuals that would lead to institutional commitment and a long-term effort to determine what might happen if professionals in education and educators in medicine joined forces. An independent observer of the midcentury scene in higher education might have thought the University of Buffalo an unlikely site for this amalgam to appear. But that is where it happened, for reasons that the next chapter may make clear.

BUFFALO:
IN THE BEGINNING . . .

2

The beginning was a mild-mannered pediatrician turned pharmacologist. Edward Bridge had already established a firm reputation as a clinician and investigator at the Johns Hopkins School of Medicine before joining the University of Buffalo faculty and the Children's Hospital staff in 1945. His professional interests were primarily in the pathologic physiology, clinical manifestations, and functional disabilities of children with convulsive disorders. By 1948 he had increasingly confined this work to the laboratory rather than the clinic; thus when an opportunity was offered to shift from pediatrics to pharmacology he grasped it.

In the new departmental setting there was far greater opportunity than in the old to see what happened to students during the early years of their medical education, and Bridge was troubled by what he saw. At a later time he described it in this now familiar way:

Students come to a medical school eager to learn, motivated strongly, and with unusually high average abilities as measured in terms of college achievement. They approach their new field with vigor and determination and also with considerable anxiety and fear. The large majority who have concentrated at college in the fields of natural science, find their experience in physics and chemistry has little if any relationship to the work they pursue. Advanced work in the field of biology helps somewhat in easing the pressure through anatomy, but in spite of this the complexities of the human body rapidly assume discouraging proportions to the new student. Within 2-4 weeks he feels overpowered, knows he cannot possibly absorb all the material described in Gray's *Anatomy,* but feels equally sure that if the final examination covers all the materials presented to him through lectures, demonstrations, laboratory dissections and quiz sections, he is likely to fail at the very outset of a hoped-for career. The advisor now finds the student in a state of confusion, sometimes amounting to near panic, wondering what to study, how to proportion his time, what is important, and usually ending up with how to pass the examinations and get on to the next hurdle. Furthermore, in this state of confusion the student finds that study habits which were held in high esteem in arts college are now useless. What place is there for thinking, reasoning, evaluating, philosophizing, when presented with the necessity of learning innumerable facts of anatomical structure? Ability to learn by rote memory, to retain facts, and to recall terms and geographical relationships become the main tools of existence. Certain types of mind adapt to such demands readily, and during the second month the pressure eases somewhat on these students. For the others, the difficulties become a life-or-death struggle with no prospect of a let-up until they have passed the final examination by fair means or foul. One might ask at this point if accomplishment in such a setting and the discipline of such a program have a relationship to the goals of medical education or to the type of person who is likely to become the successful practitioner . . . One might ask too if the present admission requirements and standards really bring to the medical schools the type of person most likely to become successful in a profession where physiological function and human relationships constitute the fundamental bases. And finally, does the present order of courses, which separates the entering student so sharply from the motivation toward human beings which brought him into the medical field, constitute an essential sequence in the curriculum?[1]

Such questions caused Bridge to think increasingly about the nature of medical school programs, to contemplate other approaches that might be used, and to talk with many people about these problems. One of those he consulted was Dr. Lester Evans, another erstwhile pediatrician and now an executive of the Commonwealth Fund.

Lester Evans is surely one of the unsung heroes in the evolution of medical education during the mid-twentieth century. His interest in seeking out promising ideas and people, his skill in encouraging the exploration of unorthodox alternatives, and his influence on the thinking of Commonwealth Fund staff and board members was felt widely in the design and support of programs that became contemporary models of educational innovation in medicine. Certainly included among the most significant of these would be the comprehensive medical care teaching project at the University of Colorado, the curriculum revision at Western Reserve University, the general medical clinic program at Cornell Medical School, and the sociologic study of medical education carried out by Robert Merton and his associates in the Bureau of Applied Social Research at Columbia University.

Considering Evans' reputation, it is not unexpected that his advice would at some point be sought by a man with Bridge's concerns. During the early months of 1950 they had several conversations, the ultimate outcome of which is probably captured most succinctly in Evans' personal file: "[Bridge] asked what a School like Buffalo might do . . . to arouse an interest in medical education among the faculty. I suggested that they might simply divide the freshman class into small groups and pick from any place in the faculty where they could find them good young teachers who would be interested in meeting with these groups of freshman students once every two weeks." The idea must have seemed reasonable, because the spring and early summer of that year at Buffalo were filled with informal meetings between Edward Bridge and physicians he identified as potential participants in such a program. By September he had convinced administration and faculty that the idea was worthwhile. I was one of fifteen Young Turks he recruited to mount the elective offering, the purpose of which was simply put: (1) to provide opportunities for the students to talk without inhibitions regarding themselves, their interests, and the medical curriculum, and (2) to expose the students to a variety of experiences illustrating the human and social aspects of disease.

The student/tutor groups were scheduled to meet for about two hours every other week. On the alternate weeks Bridge proposed that the tutors come together to discuss their observations and to consider methods of applying modern principles of education to their own instructional problems. In this way the Seminar on Medical Education began; it continued without interruption for five academic years. Before coming to an end the tutorial program and seminar series involved nearly 100 medical school faculty members.

For clinicians, teaching first-year medical students was a new and somewhat unsettling experience. Most had previously found the excitement of student-teacher interaction to come from pursuing together elusive answers to the challenging problems with which wards and clinics were filled, and from sharing with students the experience they had gained, the insights they had developed, and the findings just emerging from their own research or that of colleagues, findings that could be translated into enhanced understanding of diagnosis and disease management. Such things were clearly not possible with beginning students. Thus the start of the program was marked by a good deal of stumbling as tutors struggled to find appropriate content and format for the meetings.

During the first two months of the school year the groups met regularly, becoming acquainted with one another, with the medical school, and with the tutorial program itself. As the intensity of regular course work increased, group discussions dealt more and more with study methods, tests, and grading, as well as with interesting applications of what was being learned, particularly in gross anatomy. As the need for general orientation lessened and study pressures continued to mount, students began to exhibit growing anxiety and confusion about what was expected of them and about their ability to succeed. Despite the reassurance many gained from the tutorial group exchanges, there was growing reluctance to devote to this activity time that might be spent in more substantive study. The result was that some tutors allowed things to drift and others reduced the frequency of meetings, while a few persisted with the regular schedule. By midyear it was evident that some change would need to be made if the program was to continue. The tutors themselves wanted it to go on not only because of the insights they were gaining from these regular encounters with beginning students but also because of a growing conviction that a close relationship with the profession for which they were preparing was useful from the moment students embarked on their medical education. At this point it was agreed that the general discussions of medicine and education that had characterized most of the previous meetings would be replaced by encounters with patients and practitioners, visits to hospitals and physicians' offices, and observation of surgical and obstetrical procedures, among other things. A quickening excitement and satisfaction was soon evident among students and tutors alike.

In retrospect this shift in focus seems obvious, but in 1950 the introduction of direct and personal clinical experience for beginning students was still a daring deviation from the mode. It was probably inevitable, as word of what was being done leaked out, that reaction would set in. It was especially intense among those who believed that there was barely enough time during the first year to deal effectively with the most basic preclinical sciences, and that such seductive entertainment simply distracted students from more important academic tasks.

Bolstered by a conviction that the work of medicine was to deal with people, not with academic content alone, and encouraged by some of the educational principles to which they were being exposed in the seminar, the small band of tutors under Bridge's leadership and with the Dean's encouragement persisted in their work. By year's end they felt it justifiable to conclude:

> The overall success of this year's program and the uniqueness of the study should leave no doubt as to the desirability of continuation. Throughout medical schools as a whole little attention has been given to the transitional problems of first-year medical students or toward the values and deficiencies in the first-year curriculum. Yet in spite of a relatively inefficient trial and error method, a clearer insight into the educational problems of this period has been obtained. With the fresh program formulated out of the experiences of the present year the success . . . should be greater next year, and policies may well evolve which could help to lay a foundation for more effective medical education everywhere.[2]

The conclusion may have been insupportable and the goal over-ambitious, but the enthusiasm of innovators is rarely tempered by judicious balance.

The medical school administration and faculty leadership were probably not convinced that great things were being accomplished, but on the other hand, neither did they feel that damage was being done. In 1951-52 the program was expanded to allow the original tutors to follow their students into the second year, while a new group was recruited for entering freshmen. Because of a personal preference to remain with beginning students, I accepted the responsibility of organizing and operating that portion of the program. It was an unusual opportunity — as well as a frightening challenge — for a very junior faculty member.

For the next five years, bedside teaching provided a central theme for this introductory program. What began as an informal semielective experience evolved into a formal offering called Introduction to Medicine. It provided a much-needed opportunity for students to gain some feeling for the relevance of what they were studying in the first-year courses to the career for which they were preparing. It was an important addition to the curriculum since the basic sciences often seemed little more than formal academic exercises at best, or initiation rites at worst. The Young Turks seemed to have won their battle and were pleased when an account of what they had done was published in a paper entitled "Bedside Teaching for First Year Students."[3] Although the publication was useful as a concise description of course organization, content, and outcome, it may have been even more informative in setting out the educational issues that provoked profound anxiety among some faculty groups and high hope among others. For it is undeniable that in the beginning there was real fear that these early clinical experiences would lessen student interest in basic science, or would create among them an unjustified confidence in their ability to deal with clinical problems independently. Although such fears proved to be unfounded, they were not unique to a medical school faculty; neither were the hopes. At the Massachusetts Institute of Technology, a faculty committee had also struggled with this issue. The conclusion that had been reached in Buffalo was not unlike the one that came out of Cambridge:

> We recognize difficulties in using professional methods and materials in the early undergraduate years when the emphasis must be on the mastery of fundamental skills and basic principles . . . But the professional spirit, the pervasive atmosphere of relevance to the outside world, the insistence on active participation by the learner rather than passive absorption, the reluctance to separate principle and practice, the belief that abstract concepts are often best taught through their applications, together provide a key to the revitalization of our instruction in all fields.[4]

Introduction to Medicine also brought home another truth. First-year students, untouched by any demand to conform to a predetermined outline for a medical history, brought to their conversations with patients a refreshing naiveté and a revealing point of view. These students were very likely to inquire into a patient's background, environment, and occupation, since these things were familiar whereas disease patterns were still unknown. They often brought back from interviews important information that their seniors, so inescapably bound to the logical pursuit of diagnosis and management, had overlooked. They were remarkably sensitive to patients' nonmedical needs, to their comfort, and to their concerns. They were not at all the cold, quick, businesslike physicians about whom the public was beginning to complain so bitterly. It was difficult to avoid the conclusion that these qualities were being trained out of students during their medical education, and that it might be better to encourage the further development of such attitudes during the early years of study than try to recapture them in special courses later.

Introducing beginning students to such an array of clinical experiences undoubtedly represented a new thrust in educational programming, but it was also being tried in various ways by other schools such as Western Reserve and the University of Pennsylvania, which had in some respects gone even further in this direction than Buffalo. The unique element of the Buffalo program was the accompanying seminar for tutors. In these gatherings the teaching group exchanged reports of successful and unsuccessful meetings with students, debated institutional organization and policy, and heard each other out on favorite issues of teaching methods, curriculum organization, or examination systems. As in many other schools, much of the discussion about these questions was based more on strongly held opinion than on firmly established fact, but this forum for ventilation and exchange also provided a setting for the introduction of new ideas. And in planning these seminars Bridge made the best possible use of that opportunity. Knowing the concerns of his constituency, he introduced resource persons drawn from other university divisions, experts who were professionally qualified to speak authoritatively about such matters as student selection, student evaluation, student study habits, the nature of learning, and the use and abuse of laboratory teaching. These contributors included, among others, professors of education, psychology, sociology, and English; the dean of liberal arts and the dean of education; a social worker; the University director of admissions; the president of a state teachers' college; and even the chancellor of the University of Buffalo.

As the paucity of their own knowledge about the process of education began to dawn upon these medical teachers, the authority with which they spoke of things known only dimly began to abate. Some even began a program of personal study to shore up their obvious deficiencies. But great care was exercised to maintain the focus of the seminar on the real educational problems they faced in order to avoid any suspicion that it was a preplanned course of instruction. There was also an effort to shift direction from time to time, to use the ninety minutes as an avenue into worlds less familiar, such as the day William Carlos Williams joined the group to share his perceptions of what patients need from their doctors—and to read some of his poetry.

It was through such experiences that the group gained a sense of cohesion and common purpose. They also gained some sense of the value of what they were doing, more through nonverbal signals than through formal words of commendation. The fact that the Dean made his office/conference room available for the meetings and often took part in the discussions himself carried an important message to the faculty at large as well as to the participants themselves.

Stockton Kimball did not project the appearance or the general demeanor of a dean. Although he was sometimes the victim of cruel caricature, his position as the scion of a distinguished Buffalo family, his personal integrity and invariable good humor, his preference for persuasion rather than dictation, his general scholarship and unquestioned fairness combined to make him a man for whom there was general affection and widespread regard. His tolerance of difference and his encouragement of divergent thinking by even the most junior faculty members created an atmosphere in which innovation could be assured a hearing and an opportunity for testing. Kimball's personal involvement in the movement of Young Turks among his faculty was an incomparable advantage.

It was the spirit of openness and readiness to explore new avenues fostered by this dean that made the University of Buffalo School of Medicine such an exciting place to be in the early fifties. Edward Bridge faithfully documented many of these activities in an annual report which no one asked him to produce but which created a sense of institutional pride each time it appeared. One of these programs was his particular joy: the replacement of conventional and cookbook laboratory exercises with individual study projects. His own Department of Pharmacology provided the first opportunity for students to undertake such work, but eventually sixteen different departments or divisions became intimately involved in this effort to foster student initiative, to satisfy individual curiosity, and to reward critical inquiry rather than parrot-like responses.

Bridge was also involved in other educational explorations, such as the effort to assure student participation in educational planning (which is commonplace today but was widely regarded as near heretical in 1950), or the renovation of an examination system that seemed more often to demand student conformity than to assess achievement of specified educational goals. Although the words were missing then, the music was that of what we now know as formative and summative evaluation. To cite another example, when the medical school moved from a central city location to the University campus, Bridge became the leader of an early effort to establish an integrated continuum of premedical and medical sciences that would assure both breadth and depth of education in a manner that emphasized the wholeness of prescribed learning rather than the separateness of its parts.

Bridge also found time to continue his exploration of new ideas and potential sources of stimulus and substance outside the University of Buffalo. During one trip to the Midwest he spent some time at the University of Chicago with Benjamin Bloom, who independently suggested the kind of collaborative study between professionals in education and those in medicine that was then in the process of gestation at Buffalo. It was welcome encouragement from one who is today a major figure in the world of education.

The spirit of innovation that was made possible by the quiet leadership of Stockton Kimball and fostered by the energy of Edward Bridge was summarized in a final paragraph of the 1951-52 report on experiments in medical education at Buffalo:

Throughout the country there is a growing discontent with the organization under which education, both undergraduate and professional, now operates. The emphasis on technical proficiency derived from books and lectures is receding in the face of developments which lay more stress on the individual and make use of active participation and experience as media for growth and maturation. There is also a growing realization that progress in the physical sciences must be counterbalanced by corresponding changes in the area of human relations and community living if society is to move forward smoothly. Experiments are in progress in at least 12 medical schools and many more colleges are seeking ways and means of making the educational program a vital and meaningful adventure. The University of Buffalo and the Niagara Frontier offer ample opportunities for such developments. The use we make of them will determine our place in the field of education in the era that lies ahead.[5]

The continuing seminar in medical education was one of the ways in which that opportunity was exploited. Among all the resource persons encountered there, the one whose message had the most profound and persistent effect was certainly Nathaniel Cantor, professor of sociology and anthropology. We first met this man, whose interest in the process of learning spanned a professional lifetime, in December 1950. Cantor had been much influenced by the work of Carl Rogers, and the seemingly structureless format he introduced into the medical education seminar shook participants who were trained in the most structured of settings. Cantor's ideas about the inextricable mixture of emotional, physical, and intellectual elements in learning, his personal performance as a seminar leader, and his matchless illustrations of the difference between what we commonly do as teachers and what is required to facilitate learning had great impact. In the course of a ninety-minute meeting not all participants were convinced, but at its conclusion none was quite as comfortable as he had been before the seminar began about what he was doing to students.

Despite the immediate effect seminar members were apparently not really ready for this message, since three years passed before Cantor was invited to return in October 1953. Once more he succeeded in shaking the seminar group, challenging some of their most jealously held views about the nature of education as well as the roles of teachers and students in that transaction. But this time there was a difference. Some of us had now worked for three years in the tutorial program and had been forced to acknowledge one inescapable fact: deficiencies that students identified in the implementation of Introduction to Medicine stemmed not from concept, which was uniformly applauded, but from teacher performance, which was frequently found wanting. The time had come to do something more than talk. We needed to become more nearly professionals in education than simply devoted amateurs.

Because of the effect he had already produced in the course of two brief encounters, Nathanial Cantor seemed a logical person to lead the group a little further. He agreed to do so, and thus began an unforgettable experience that was later described as an "Adventure in Pedagogy."[6] The adventure occurred over a period of 20 hours—ten 2-hour seminars at weekly intervals. The purported text was Cantor's book, *The Teaching* ⇌ *Learning Process,*[7] but the real text was our own experience as teachers and learners, drawn out and examined under Cantor's masterful leadership. It is impossible to capture the full flavor of this interaction in a few paragraphs, but the experience was of such pivotal importance in further evolution of the Buffalo program that this account would be incomplete without some attempt to summarize at least its substance.

One of the early things the group came to accept was that people learn what they want to learn. A simple but revealing example might be the medical student who has difficulty recalling the sequence of the Krebs cycle but can recite without hesitation the batting average of every player in the major leagues and the telephone numbers of twelve attractive girls. Teachers cannot call him stupid, since the Admissions Committee has ruled out this possibility, but they may be inclined to question his motivation, since anyone who wants to be a physician should also want this basic bit of biochemical knowledge. This judgment relieves a faculty member of further responsibility but gives little help to the struggling student. Furthermore, such an action implies that teachers can decide what students should *want* to learn, which is surely unrealistic, if not absurd. The challenging task is to help students want what they need. Any teacher who establishes some meaningful link between learning the Krebs cycle and effective performance as a physician will find it difficult to stop medical students from absorbing that knowledge eagerly and enthusiastically. Motivation relates not only to the distant goal but to each of the stepping-stones that lead there.

Closely related was the principle that knowledge and learning are different. Medical faculties place a premium on the accumulation of factual information by using examinations that reward immediate recall of facts as an effective prod. This is done in the belief that education is an intellectual exercise, ignoring a repeatedly demonstrated fact that most of what is learned in this way has a very short half-life. Significant learning is clearly an emotional as well as an intellectual experience. The things we retain are those that kindle a spark, arouse curiosity, or incite anger, disagreement, or laughter. And for each of us these things may be different, since learning is also a very personal process.

The group also soon recognized that true learning implies change. In the course of ten seminars it became painfully evident that the first law of thermodynamics, the law of inertia, applies with equal force to learning. A large part of the discussion time was spent in defending our established positions on educational practice and resisting personal change by the classic methods we had seen our students use: tardiness, failure to complete assignments, shifting the focus of discussion when it came close to tender spots, obscuring issues by vagueness, and indulging in hair-splitting, self-deception, and hostility. But progress and change did take place, in a direction and at a pace acceptable to the group, under the skilled guidance of a leader who made no value judgment about these tactics but simply accepted them as an inevitable part of the learning.

Finally, we had to acknowledge that true learning requires freedom. This concept did not imply educational anarchy, in which students did only what they wanted to do, but rather freedom from arbitrary external power. Most medical education seems to lack this quality; it is content- and examination-oriented, providing freedom for students to grow in only one way. Those who do what they are told and give back the "official pitch" when called upon are labeled good students, while those who analyze and challenge and accept nothing without supporting evidence are commonly regarded as annoying at least, and possibly in need of therapy. Encouragement of independent thinking, which is what higher education is said to be about, makes life considerably more trying for a faculty. Traditional teaching is relatively easy, but helping students to learn is an exhausting occupation.

The basic responsibility of a teacher finally became obvious to the group. It is rooted in the fundamental respect for individuals that allows each student the freedom to be different, that encourages in all a desire to learn rather than to know, that manifests itself as an honest effort to understand students rather than to judge them. Although the lesson has not always been learned, it should be easier for a physician-teacher than for almost any other. A physician's basic work is to provide a professional service to patients, one aimed at understanding their problems and helping them to find solutions. There is no moral judgment of the illness a patient presents, and no loss of self-esteem if advice is ignored or the disease fails to respond to the best therapeutic intervention. It is just such a professional service that teachers owe to students; anything less is a fraud.

Nearly twenty-five years later, seven of the participants in that experience responded to my inquiry about whether it had influenced their attitudes about education or their performance as teachers. The response was uniformly and resoundingly affirmative. It was perhaps expressed most feelingly by John Boylan, an internist-physiologist, who wrote: "I'm sure I was permanently imprinted by Nat Cantor and have never thought the same again about students, or learning, or education. He was unique, a once-in-a-lifetime experience." My own long-term assessment was summarized in a foreword written for the 1972 reprinting of one of Cantor's most influential books.[8] The heart of the message was that he had helped all of us take a giant step toward the goal Comenius sought in the fifteenth century: a method of instruction by which teachers may teach less, but learners may learn more.

In this age when literally scores of teachers in dozens of medical schools have undergone such an experience, it may be difficult to picture the controversy this program aroused at the time. Not only was the content dismissed as trivial by a substantial number of Buffalo medical faculty members, but also the involvement of an "educationalist" was regarded by many as a violation of our professional dignity. Those views were perhaps best illustrated by the response of an aggressive surgeon to my comment that professional educators seemed to exhibit greater humility about understanding the educational process than we did. "They have more to be humble about!" he said without hesitation—and without question.

There were, of course, those who took quiet pride in the national recognition that accompanied the publication of "Adventure in Pedagogy." But antagonists were overjoyed when Professor R. A. Lyman, chairman of the Department of Zoology and director of the Student Health Service at Idaho State College, attacked the educational concepts embodied there in a special article that appeared nine months later in the *New England Journal of Medicine*. Using the title "Disaster in Pedagogy," Lyman called the adventure "A skillful blending of valid, though trite, criticism of medical education, and the sheer nonsense that composes the educationalists' party line." He concluded with what some might describe as another party line: "No one denies that medical education can be and should be improved. The question is, are medical educators going to set about it in a rational fashion with efforts to restore the discipline of learning throughout the entire educational system? Or will they attempt it by encouraging in medical education the same practices and philosophy that have made the high schools of the country a national disgrace?"[9] But this national fallout was now too late to do more than arouse further interest in the expanded program that had by then been firmly established.

Few things heighten aspiration more than success. Certainly the promising outcome of these teaching-learning seminars was an important factor in the development of a more elaborate training program for medical teachers. The outline of that vision was still seen only dimly, but the general form was that of a year-long faculty fellowship, a work/study program designed to provide the philosophic base, the cognitive structure, and the technical skills that should characterize a professional faculty member.

Five broad areas seemed appropriate for study in sufficient depth to assure both perspective and understanding. First, of course, was the *teaching-learning process* with which so much useful experience had already been gained. The second element was the *nature of the medical student,* since learning must begin where students are (not where faculty might wish they were), and it is important for teachers to have a clear view of the procedures by which students are selected, the individual differences among them, and the motivations as well as the social and cultural factors that influence their response to educational programs. The third topic was the *materials and methods of instruction,* both the varied means by which learning of different kinds can be facilitated (or impeded) and the skills required to use these tools effectively. The fourth area was *evaluation* of students and programs, the basic principles of assessment and the techniques that may be employed to gather sound data both for facilitating learning and for judging the outcome. The fifth component dealt with the general *background of higher education*—the evolution of educational ideas, of contemporary trends, of how medical education fits into the overall pattern of academic organization and values.

The work portion of the program was seen as an opportunity for faculty Fellows to translate into practice, and to test in the classroom, laboratory, clinic, or ward, the principles that had emerged from their systematic studies. Whether these topics were most useful for dealing with problems that medical teachers face, whether their careful consideration could modify the conventional perception of a teacher's role, and whether such study would be reflected in changed teaching practices remained to be confirmed empirically. Thus an evaluation plan was also incorporated into the preliminary five-year projection.

Up to this point the work had been carried on without any special budget, supported only by the interest of faculty members whose academic responsibilities were for other things. A more ambitious program would clearly require external funding as well as internal backing. Dean Kimball's participation in the Cantor seminar proved to be a vital factor in winning both, for his endorsement was seen as the product of personal experience, not of intellectual assent alone.

Although initiative came from the School of Medicine, a program of this kind could not be mounted without the active participation of other university divisions, and particularly that of the School of Education. Fortunately the dean of that unit, Robert Fisk, was not daunted by unorthodox proposals, although he was startled by the request. Schools of education are not often confronted by appeals for assistance from other parts of the higher education community, and in this instance Fisk was not sure that his faculty knew enough about medical education to be helpful. Nonetheless it struck him as an exciting challenge, one that was well worth pursuing. He identified two younger members of his faculty as the most likely contributors to such collaboration and suggested that I attempt to arouse their interest. It was not difficult to do so, and in this way Stephen Abramson and Robert Harnack, important figures in the next stage of program development, became involved in what proved for one of them to be the start of a new career.

With support from the School of Education assured and endorsement from the School of Liberal Arts and university administration also won, it was now necessary to gain the sanction of leaders in the medical school. Interviews with department heads and other significant figures in that setting were not always as easy or as positive as those carried out in other parts of the university, where the response had without exception been one of high interest. However, by early spring of 1954 a majority of medical school department heads had agreed to support such a program and the others expressed willingness to cooperate, although without any great enthusiasm for doing so.

On the basis of this degree of acceptance a broadly representative university group was invited to serve in an advisory capacity as a program proposal was developed in greater detail. This committee included, in addition to Dean Kimball and Dean Fisk, Stephen Abrahamson, Vice Chancellor Lester Anderson, Nathaniel Cantor, Associate Dean (of Liberal Arts) Richard Drake, and the Distinguished Professor of Bacteriology Ernest Witebsky. Their initial meeting was held in May, and the first advice they offered was to change the proposed program title from Project in Medical Teacher Training to Project in Medical Education. It was good advice, as were the more substantive suggestions offered as the work evolved. Now, however, their principal action was review, and approval with minor modifications, of a concrete proposal I had distributed in draft form prior to the meeting. With this endorsement in hand a presentation was made two weeks later to the School of Medicine Executive Committee, where approval was moved by the professor of surgery and passed without dissent.

Now the search for funds began. The first feeler went out to the Kellogg Foundation, where Matthew Kinde was sufficiently intrigued by the preliminary description of what was proposed to spend a June day in Buffalo talking to program planners, prior participants, and members of the Advisory Committee. What he heard heightened his initial interest. He pointed out, however, that this was an entirely new approach to medical education, one that might not warrant a financial commitment since the Foundation had already invested heavily in other areas. Later review by other members of the Kellogg staff confirmed the hint Kinde had given. In September, visits to the Rockefeller Foundation, the Fund for the Advancement of Education, and the Hartford Foundation produced polite expressions of interest but also of regret that what was being proposed did not match current program priorities. Only Lester Evans at the Commonwealth Fund was really encouraging, although he used the carefully chosen words any first-rate foundation executive employs to avoid misinterpretation or unjustified hopes. However, the notes he filed following my visit give an interesting independent assessment of what was then taking place at the University of Buffalo:

About two years ago the University asked the fund for a small grant . . . but at that time we felt the University really was not ready to go as far as it wanted and we had some doubts about the quality of the Medical School leadership. Miller was, therefore, somewhat apologetic when he came in this time, saying he did not know how we felt about Buffalo but hoped that our attitude was more favorable than in the past. I immediately stated that our attitude had not been unfavorable but rather that in our judgment, and with the commitments we then had pending, Buffalo did not seem to offer the opportunity we wanted. I also hurriedly explained that I had seen no university or medical school faculty go as far as the Buffalo group has now gone on its own without assistance . . .

My interpretation of this proposal at the moment is something like this. That heretofore we have been asked to assist medical education by approaching it through study and rearrangement of the curriculum, for example, Western Reserve; the reorganization of subject matter, for example, Harvard basic science; the demonstration of a new type of patient care, for example, Cornell. But, only recently has there been any talk, even among these groups, as to the necessity of doing something about the teachers themselves. Now Buffalo says they would like to concentrate on teacher training, so to speak, in the belief, from what they have seen over the last five years, that medical school teachers thoroughly familiar with such topics as listed in their proposal would quite automatically change course structure, course content, sequence of educational experience, and so forth to meet what they will have come to recognize as the student's educational or learning needs . . .

Even though there is much for the University to do in working out the detail and implementation of their proposal and much for us to do in appreciating this approach to the study of medical education, I hope that we can, if the University so indicates, continue discussion with them.

The cautious expression of interest that Evans had given led Dean Kimball to send him a formal invitation to visit the university again in order to discuss further what had been achieved and what was being proposed. This invitation apparently precipitated a Commonwealth Fund staff review of the distant background and more recent exchanges with Buffalo and produced a flurry of internal notes that suggested some ambivalence ("Why can't this sort of thing be done after hours rather than requiring additional staff?" "Why is this brought to us by an Assistant Professor of Medicine rather than the Dean?"). But there was general agreement that the proposal deserved further consideration ("I do not know of any graduate or professional school which has systematically assisted new, young faculty members in understanding the educational process better, and in becoming better teachers . . .").

Responsibility for making an initial site visit in November was given to Charles Warren, whose critical analysis, objective observations, and constructive suggestions ultimately contributed so greatly to the work then being proposed. But he did not begin with unbridled enthusiasm. In fact, Warren's field notes indicate clearly that he started out in a distinctly ambivalent frame of mind. Two days of meetings with those most directly involved, as well as other faculty members and administrators, apparently dispelled that feeling. On returning to New York he reported that there was such promise in the Buffalo ideas and setting that if a formal request for support was submitted it should be pursued.

Shortly before Christmas the advisory committee, which had been meeting regularly during the fall term, endorsed the draft of a formal proposal. A refined document was approved by the medical school executive committee in January. On February 1, 1955, Chancellor Clifford C. Furnas submitted the proposal to the Commonwealth Fund. The key paragraph of his covering letter read:

> The School of Medicine has taken a position of leadership in the development of this project and the immediate focus is upon education within that school . . . It is important to point out, however, that this program, which has been nearly a year in development, reflects the mutual and complementary interests of several University divisions in a problem which has relevance to all. It can also claim the full backing of the University administration.

The plan submitted was essentially an elaboration and amplification of the original prospectus. In order to round out the story a summary of the final specifications must certainly be included here, beginning with program objectives:

1. To determine the importance to the education of medical students of an increased awareness among medical teachers of fundamental educational principles.

2. To determine the feasibility of a continuing cooperative effort between a school of medicine and other university divisions in the development of more effective teachers in medicine.
3. To assess the effect of changes in mode of instruction that may result from this teacher training program upon medical student learning.
4. To determine the practicality of such an approach to the educational problems of medical schools.

During each of the four years following an initial year of detailed program planning, a minimum of four University of Buffalo School of Medicine faculty members and four visiting faculty from comparable departments would take part in the work/study program. All were to be selected on the basis of interest in teaching as well as competence in their discipline. The local faculty members would be relieved of a part of their regular responsibilities, while visiting counterparts would be integrated into departmental work to fill the gap thus created. At the end of each year local and visiting Fellows would return to their regular activities and home settings. By this means the influence on other schools of those who had devoted a full year to the intensive study and application of educational science to instructional programs in medicine could also be studied. If the effect of this training was sufficiently promising, an increase in the number of participants, not to exceed sixteen, might be considered for the last two project years.

Faculty Fellows would be expected to devote themselves fully to the year-long work/study program, which was planned to begin two weeks before the regular academic year got under way. During the first of these weeks an introductory seminar on one of the five proposed topics would be held each afternoon. In the morning visiting faculty would be introduced by their local counterparts to other members of the department and given an opportunity to familiarize themselves with departmental facilities, instructional programs, and their own academic assignment for the year. The second week would be devoted to an intensive consideration of the teaching-learnng process in a two-hour seminar each morning and afternoon. For the remainder of the year one half of each day would be given to regular departmental activities, the other half to independent study and seminar discussion of the selected educational topics.

Techniques for evaluating the influence of the program on participants, students, colleagues, and educational programs would be developed during the initial planning year. It was anticipated that both subjective impressions and objective data could be gathered through such methods as critical review of the experience at regular intervals by participants and staff, departmental appraisal of the program's effect on instruction and students, more systematic assessment of attitude and learning changes through questionnaires and other testing devices, and later follow-up of both local and visiting participants as well as their students and colleagues.

The response of the Commonwealth Fund was prompt and positive. Two weeks after the proposal was submitted, Warren suggested that a formal site visit be made in March to review in detail the program and the setting. He would be accompanied by John Eberhart, another staff member to whom the Project in Medical Education came to owe a great debt for wise counsel as well as continuing support. But in February no one knew how things would turn out, and there was an understandable tension in the air.

Warren and Eberhart spent three days in Buffalo. What they saw and heard, the interpretations and judgments they made, were spelled out in a set of field notes, now in the Commonwealth Fund archives. Although these comments may have the greatest interest for those who were intimately involved, they are so informative and revealing that extensive quotation seems justified to give contemporary readers, who live in a very different climate of opinion, a better understanding of how things were in 1955:

> This is a unique proposal, something quite different from anything in the field of medical education that we have been asked to consider previously. Its novelty, of course, doesn't of itself make the program good, but it is my feeling that the project is both novel *and* good. I base this on the following considerations:
>
> 1. The project is essentially a study of medical education, plus some experimenting with it, as a joint undertaking by medical and non-medical professionals. Including the latter in the manner proposed is an excellent idea since it is bound to bring new thinking into the field. Yet these contributions from education, sociology, and psychology will meet the day-to-day discussion, criticism, and in some instances, actual testing by medical school faculty members. The latter will, of course, be making contributions themselves. The give-and-take that will inevitably result should be an almost ideal testing ground for new approaches to medical education.

2. Having the focus on the learning process to the extent indicated in the prospectus is also a good idea. It is obviously an important matter that has hitherto received far too little attention in medical schools and never the systematic study that is proposed here.

3. While the ideas behind the proposal are attractive and seem sound, the project's most important asset, so it seems to me, is the quality of the people involved . . . The whole group of them are keen and highly motivated; it can be counted on to get the maximum out of the particular approaches they are using.

4. The fact that major curricular changes are not proposed at the outset should not be viewed with misgiving. This group realizes perfectly well that a good curriculum is a vital part of any educational program and they will certainly be analyzing curriculum structure to see what kinds of changes pretty much *have* to be made. But the fact that they want to start out finding out how much can be done *within* the present assignment of hours seems a perfectly sensible thing to do and one which obviously has potentialities for widespread application.

5. The program will doubtless have at least two general kinds of impact. In the first place, an activity of this magnitude and intensity cannot go on in a school like Buffalo without sensitizing pretty much the whole school to its educational program. Although the medical school participants will be in only four departments at one time, the plan is to make it a new four each year, which in three years will pretty much cover the school. Having two young people in a department that are as deeply interested in medical education as these participants will be can't help but provoke an unusually close examination of the department's educational activities.

The other general kind of impact will be on the participants, both the medical people and the others. I would doubt that anyone could spend a year in the program without its having a notable effect on his knowledge of and approach to a variety of the educational problems in medicine. The only question will be how much influence the participants from other medical schools will have on their own schools when they return.

6. The situation in which this program is to be carried out is a favorable one for the project. The University of Buffalo has the people, in and out of the medical school, to implement it, and they are strongly motivated to do so. The medical school is one that has not been outstanding in the past but in recent

years it has begun to move. The relations between the University and the medical school are good and will be greatly strengthened if the program goes into effect. There is good administrative support for the program in both areas.

7. Finally, although this is something we don't often discuss, what would happen if the Fund failed to support this project? It would be taken as a vote of lack of confidence on the part of a group who are known to be particularly interested in medical education and I doubt that other support would be found for it . . . It would largely prevent a group of highly motivated and capable people from making their optimum contribution to medical education. I think that the latter, as well as the individuals concerned, would feel the loss.

Putting it most simply, I view this project as potentially contributing importantly to medical education. It is almost a "natural" for the Fund at this time and I recommend its support in line with the above budget.

Of course, no such frank observations and conclusions were revealed in the course of the site visit. Instead the planners were asked to spell out in greater detail several elements of the proposal (and particularly the part that dealt with evaluation); they were offered encouragement but were also reminded that it carried no implication of Fund commitment; and they were told that the proposal would probably be acted upon by the board of directors at their May meeting. Then the waiting began.

The first blow came in April when John Eberhart called to say that it had not been possible to prepare the necessary supporting documents for board review in May, but that the proposal would probably be dealt with by the board's Executive Committee in July. Equally distressing was his report that the Fund staff could not recommend support for the extensive evaluation study that had been proposed but would suggest a more simplified and less costly narrative account of progress and outcome. Swallowing hard, the planning group decided not to contest this decision but to do what could be done within the limits suggested if the program were supported.

The second blow came in July when Eberhart wrote to say that the executive committee had decided the proposal should be reviewed by the full board of directors before final action was taken. Unfortunately, the next board meeting would not be held until November.

Finally, on November 18, 1955, Malcolm Aldrich, President of the Commonwealth Fund, informed Chancellor Furnas that the Fund had appropriated $131,400 to support the Project in Medical Education for the period from December 1, 1955, to August 31, 1958. The Chancellor responded in characteristic fashion by noting: "Even though it is said to be more blessed to give than to receive, I wish to assure you that the pleasure you expressed in your letter of November 18th was small compared to our own by the news of your grant . . ."

At last, the project was under way.

BUFFALO: THE PROJECT
IN MEDICAL EDUCATION

3

With support now assured, planning was accelerated since the work initially projected for a full year had to be compressed into nine months. The major tasks were three in number: (1) preparation of seminar content and leaders; (2) recruitment of participants; and (3) development of an evaluation mechanism that could be implemented within the established limits of personnel and funds.

PREPARATION

While awaiting Commonwealth Fund action on the request for support, the program advisory committee had continued to meet and to make preliminary policy decisions in anticipation of a favorable response. One of the most important agreements they reached was to have joint leadership in each of the five seminar series. With responsibility shared by medical and educational professionals, a model of mutual understanding and support would be established and the desired balance between academic soundness and pragmatic utility would be assured. Most of the potential leaders had already taken part in the preliminary discussions, but now a final commitment of time and energy was required. Assignments were finally made in this way:

1. *The teaching-learning process.* Nathaniel Cantor, chairman of the Department of Sociology and Anthropology, had long been identified with the medical education program; his earlier contributions have already been described. Phillip Wels, instructor in surgery, had been a participant in the original faculty seminar on learning; and as a tutor in Introduction to Medicine he had put to

the test of practice the principles highlighted during that seminar experience.

2. *The nature of the medical student.* Ira Cohen, assistant professor of psychology, was acting head of the psychology clinic, where he had gained valuable experience in dealing with student problems as well as in working with other health professionals. Harold Graser, instructor in psychiatry in the School of Medicine, was also a professorial lecturer in both the College of Arts and Sciences and the School of Social Work. His familiarity with medical student problems, as well as his interdisciplinary orientation, identified him as a particularly valuable contributor to this seminar.

3. *Evaluation.* Stephen Abrahamson, associate professor of education and director of the Educational Research Center in the College of Education, was also a member of the project advisory committee. Ivan Bunnell, assistant professor of physiology and of medicine and director of the Buffalo General Hospital outpatient department, had been a participant in the original seminar on medical education and in the subsequent teaching-learning seminars conducted by Nathaniel Cantor.

4. *Communication, including techniques of instruction.* Robert Harnack, associate professor of education and a specialist in curriculum and instruction, was an important contributor to the discussions that led to formulation of the proposal to the Commonwealth Fund. I was the second member of this team. As an assistant professor of medicine, director of house staff education at the Buffalo General Hospital, and now Coordinator of the Project in Medical Education, my interests were shifting steadily from problems of water and electrolyte metabolism to those of educating physicians.

5. *The evolution of higher, particularly of medical, education.* Lester Anderson, vice chancellor for educational affairs and professor of higher education, had already made a significant contribution to planning the project as a member of the advisory committee and seemed to be an ideal professional educational resource for this seminar. His pairing with Edward Bridge, professor of pharmacology, was a particularly happy one. However, during the preparatory period Bridge was persuaded to head the newly established, AID-supported affiliation between the University of Buffalo and the University of Paraguay, which took him from Buffalo to Asunción. Joseph Macmanus, associate clinical professor of surgery and an in-

formal student of educational philosophy, agreed to fill the role
from which Bridge had to withdraw. During the second program
year this responsibiltiy was carried out by Dean Stockton Kimball.

The worth of joint medical and nonmedical seminar leadership
was demonstrated again and again during the late winter, spring,
and summer. As they struggled to reach agreement on seminar organization, content, and implementation, many of the pairs of
leaders spent long hours together observing medical school lectures,
laboratory exercises, ward and clinic teaching. The educators were
seeing such instruction for the first time; the physicians were seeing
it anew through the eyes of colleagues who were more concerned
about educational process than with subject matter content. Each
team had an opportunity to engage in such observational study not
only at Buffalo but also in one or more other medical schools where
they thought some special insight might be gained, such as Cornell,
New York University, Columbia, Rochester, and the University of
Colorado. Through such shared experiences the seminar leaders
gained new respect for one another, new perceptions of the nature
of medical education, and a heightened awareness of how their
individual competencies supplemented and complemented each
other.

It was equally important for these leaders to sustain their vision of
the project as a unified whole, not merely as five independent seminars loosely related to practical field work in medical school departments. This unitary view was facilitated by monthly meetings of the
entire group during which individual seminar planning became a
shared experience. The team building effort was climaxed by a two-
day visit to Western Reserve University, scene of the sharpest break
with educational tradition in medicine that had occurred since the
Flexnerian revolution. The searching, critical, but always good-
humored exchanges that characterized these meetings at home and
abroad succeeded beyond the most optimistic hope in welding individual leaders into an enthusiastic team in which each member felt
a sense of responsibility for the total program and not for a single
seminar series alone.

One further addition to the leadership group was proposed during the preparatory period. Because virtually all those from the
medical faculty were viewed as converts to a new way of approaching education (even in some instances as missionary zealots), it
seemed important to add someone who had not been a part of the
original group, who was seen as sound and objective, and who could

serve a neutral liaison function between the project staff and the general medical faculty and student body. Harold Brody, assistant professor of anatomy, accepted this assignment, which proved to be more symbolic than functional but was unquestionably an important symbol at the time.

RECRUITMENT

Recruitment of local faculty participants for 1956-57 began almost immediately after announcement of the Commonwealth Fund award in December; that of visiting faculty was delayed until the following February when the annual Congress on Medical Education met in Chicago. In preparation for that national search, a brief description of the project, with a covering letter from Dean Kimball, was sent to the dean of each medical school in the United States and Canada. Although no reply was required, thirty-three responded with comments ranging from simple acknowledgment to great enthusiasm for what was being proposed. Four even expressed hope that they could nominate a candidate. Personal discussion with more than a score of deans was managed during the three-day Chicago meeting. Their reaction was uniformly favorable, although many voiced reservations about the contribution professional educators could make to such a program. Several deans even described their own attempts to initiate similar work. Each of these efforts had been foiled by the educationist's inability to communicate with medical faculty members, and the experience succeeded only in arousing antagonism.

Serious questions were also raised about whether it was realistic to expect a medical faculty member to spend a full year in education, at the expense of continued productivity in basic or clinical research, especially when the academic community rarely rewards pedagogic skill. More often hinted at than verbalized was the equally troublesome question of whether there was really enough substance in the discipline of education to justify so much time in its study.

Despite these reservations, which were heard locally as often as in the national arena, interest mounted. By late winter the four participating departments at Buffalo had been identified, and by spring four local and three visiting faculty participants had been selected:

1. *Bacteriology.* Reginald Lambert, Ph.D., a graduate of the University of Buffalo, had been a member of the Department of Bacteriology for one year. Despite vigorous recruitment efforts, which continued until the program began in September, no available counterpart from another school could be found.

2. *Obstetrics and Gynecology.* Kenneth Niswander, M.D., a graduate of the University of Buffalo, had completed his specialty training at the Buffalo General Hospital. Now a part-time faculty member, Niswander had for two years served as departmental executive officer for the student teaching program. John Harkins, M.D., a graduate of the University of Toronto, was now a member of that faculty. After the year in Buffalo, he would return to Toronto to assume increased responsibility for the teaching program in his department.

3. *Pharmacology.* Dean LeSher, Ph.D., a graduate of the University of Wisconsin, had been a member of the Buffalo faculty for one year. Murray Blair, Ph.D., a graduate of Tufts University, had been a part of that medical faculty for three years. After the year in Buffalo, he would be given greater responsibility for both medical and dental courses in pharmacology at Tufts.

4. *Surgery.* Donald Becker, M.D., a graduate of the University of Pennsylvania, had recently completed a five-year surgical residency. He was now a part-time faculty member working at the Meyer Memorial Hospital in Buffalo. Robert Cordell, M.D., a graduate of Johns Hopkins School of Medicine, had just completed his surgical training at Bowman Gray School of Medicine, where he would become a full-time faculty member at the conclusion of the year in Buffalo.

One additional participant appeared from an unexpected source. A third-year medical student faced by the newly established requirement for a senior thesis selected medical education as his topic. Stimulated by reading a draft of "Adventure in Pedagogy" and excited by the proposed teacher training program, he asked for an opportunity to take part in the Project in Medical Education. After lengthy discussion with this student, with the project advisory committee, and with the school of medicine executive committee, it was finally agreed that Hilliard Jason would spend two years completing the final year of medical school so that he could also participate in the project and work simultaneously toward a doctoral degree in education. The inclusion of a perceptive student in this first round proved to be useful for both the group and the individual.

EVALUATION

In all educational development efforts, one of the most troublesome questions is that of evaluation; it was certainly true in this project. The Educational Research Center, under Stephen Abrahamson's direction, provided conceptual and technical guidance in fleshing out the initial evaluation plan, but that plan was subjected to merciless scrutiny as well as significant modification first by the advisory committee and later by the project sponsor.

The preliminary proposal pointed out that the project was designed to test the hypothesis that an increased awareness of educational principles would lead to changes in the attitudes of medical teachers toward the process of medical education and in their instructional practices. It was assumed that these attitudinal changes would result in more efficient student learning, that the instructional changes would lead to more positive attitudes among students toward their own responsibilities, and that all these changes would produce medical school graduates better prepared to function as physicians. More specifically, it was expected that the attitudinal changes among participants would occur in five broad areas: toward teaching, toward the objectives of medical education, toward the organization of subject matter, toward medical students, and toward colleagues. The specific changes in instructional practices were to be further defined in the course of program planning.

Out of these considerations emerged a plan to study (1) the attitudes and classroom performance of participants and of matched controls; (2) the attitudes and achievement of students taught by seminar participants at the University of Buffalo and of matched controls in other schools; and (3) the performance of seminar leaders (in an effort to separate the impact of content and process from that of individual charisma). Contemplated study methods included interview, log/diary, formal attitude testing, direct observation of performance, and follow-up in the home setting.

In ensuing discussions the theoretical, operational, and fiscal questions raised by such an elaborate undertaking were dealt with, and compromises acceptable to project staff, advisory committee, the Educational Research Center, and the Commonwealth Fund were ultimately achieved.

The formal procedure finally agreed upon was to be carried out in six stages:

1. At least six nonparticipant medical faculty members were to be interviewed to obtain basic information about attitudes in the five general categories noted earlier, as background for creating a structured interview schedule to be used with participants.
2. Each participant was to be interviewed before the seminars began, to gain baseline information about attitudes held at the start of their study.
3. A daily log/diary was to be completed by each participant, to gain insight into running perceptions of the program and evidence of changing attitudes if changes did occur.
4. Each participant was to be interviewed every other week, to validate interpretations of log/diary entries, to explore significant items in greater depth, and to create an opportunity for additional information to be exchanged.
5. Periodic observation was to be made of participants in their instructional activities, to determine the nature of that performance and whether changes occurred in the course of the year.
6. Anecdotal records were to be kept by seminar leaders, to document noteworthy occurrences in interaction with participants or significant changes in individual behavior.

In addition to this formal accumulation and analysis of data, an informal assessment of the program was to be attempted through the eyes of visiting medical educators. Each visitor would spend several days taking an independent sounding of what was being done and making an independent judgment of what was being achieved. This method had the additional advantage of familiarizing others with the program through personal encounter rather than written description. Their reports, if favorable, would certainly lend credibility to the worth of an effort that was not universally regarded as worthy.

Agreement on this general plan was achieved in May 1956. A detailed work plan had to be completed by September, when the program was scheduled to start. Fortunately, Abrahamson had working in his Educational Research Center a young graduate student who was attracted by the challenge of developing the methodology and who was willing to serve as the principal staff person to carry out the evaluation study. It was a happy coincidence of interest and need, for Edwin Rosinski became a significant figure not only in the project itself but also in the subsequent maturation of research in medical education as a legitimate field of study.

IMPLEMENTATION: ROUND ONE

Now the stage was set and the play was about to begin. Visiting faculty members arrived shortly after Labor Day in 1956. They were introduced by their counterparts to the departmental setting and, through social events, to the others with whom they would live and work for a year. It was thus a reasonably comfortable group that began an intensive consideration of the teaching-learning process in two 2-hour seminars each day during the week of September 17. By the end of that introduction the group members were intellectually shaken and emotionally drained, but they no longer questioned (if they ever had) that this would be a challenging and rewarding experience. The seminar schedule for the remainder of the year was far less intense (Figure 3.1). There was time for reading and reflecting as well as for talking and teaching. And there was the never-ending expectation that each individual would document what was happening. (It is probably important to note that the participants were far more faithful in keeping log/diaries than were the leaders in providing anecdotal records.)

With one exception the year evolved according to plan, but that exception was a devastating blow. About mid-October, illness overtook Nathaniel Cantor. The surgery that followed kept him out of the program until early 1957, but the vigor of his contribution was never fully restored. In Cantor's absence I joined Phil Wels in lead-

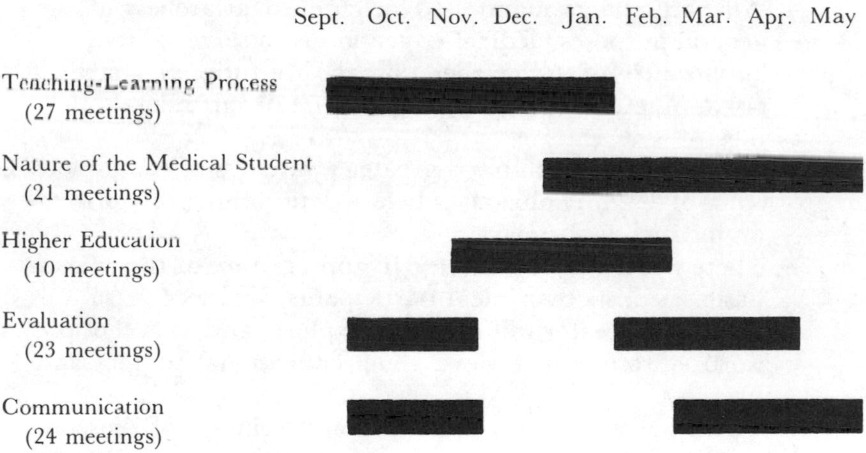

FIGURE 3.1. Seminar/workshop schedule, Project in Medical Education, 1956-57.

ing the teaching-learning seminar, but we were certainly no substitute for the master.

By June a vast quantity of information about the program had
been accumulated from participants and seminar leaders, from four
distinguished visiting medical educators, and from Commonwealth
Fund staff members who had returned for several days in the spring
to see the program in action. From each of these sources strengths as
well as weaknesses in program planning, administration, organization, and operation were identified, but all came to the same general conclusion: it had been a remarkably successful undertaking.

The most reliable findings were probably the attitudinal data
that were systematically assembled throughout the year and systematically analyzed by the Educational Research Center. Rosinski
summarized the outcome in a set of ten generalizations:

1. Participants with a decidedly one-sided point of view about
   education tended to moderate that stance.
2. All participants evidenced slowly increased awareness of the
   variety of techniques available to facilitate the teaching-
   learning exchange.
3. All participants now expressed intelligent concern for the
   appropriateness of specific techniques, whereas in the beginning they had been more inclined to condemn or con-
   done without reference to such factors as teacher skill in
   using a method, student readiness to benefit, or the extent
   to which subject matter lent itself to a given instructional
   mode.
4. All participants manifested heightened awareness of the
   general purposes medical education is to serve, and of the
   importance of using these broad institutional goals as
   points of reference in planning specific departmental offerings.
5. All participants exhibited greater awareness of the importance of defining objectives before determining the form of
   an instructional program.
6. There was a general increase in appreciation of the role of
   basic scientists by clinical participants, and vice versa.
7. There was greater willingness to explore, and to accept the
   worth of, alternative views about educational content and
   process.
8. There was a generally enhanced appreciation of the contribution to medical education that could be made by professional educators.

9. There was uniformly increased awareness of the complexity of formal education and of the teaching-learning process.
10. There was general recognition that knowledge of subject matter is an essential but insufficient criterion for the preparation or identification of a good teacher.

In 1980 these may seem like small gains, but in 1956 they were giant steps. It was particularly impressive to have these attitudes of young faculty members who had been subjected to a year-long program confirmed by senior external observers. For example, Dr. Donald Anderson, dean of the University of Rochester School of Medicine and Dentistry and a former secretary of the American Medical Association Council on Medical Education, said:

> In conclusion my estimate of the worth of the project as it has developed to date can best be expressed by stating that I would be most hopeful that some day we could have the opportunity to try a similar program.
>
> Buffalo is clearly exploring new territory in medical education and the results should be of real value to all the other schools in the United States and Canada and perhaps ultimately to schools throughout the world.

Dr. Vernon Lippard, dean of the Yale University School of Medicine, noted:

> Most men enter medical faculties with little understanding of the organization or policies of the institution with which they become associated, and of the goals of the course they are to teach, of the relation of their efforts to those of others, of the methods of communicating information or influencing attitudes, etc. . . . Conferences dealing with these and similar topics could be of great value to young instructors and would be profitable to older men, if they could be persuaded to attend. Having broken the ice, I hope that the cooperative research program will be continued indefinitely, with special emphasis on development of techniques for evaluation of instructional methods.
>
> Looking to the future, I have serious doubts as to the advisability of continuing an extensive fellowship program for a dozen young instructors, year after year, at Buffalo or elsewhere. Based on the experience gained in this experiment, however, I can see great value in the development of a syllabus or outline for a series of bi-weekly conferences over an academic year for new faculty members at any medical school.

Dr. John Cowles, assistant to the vice chancellor, Schools of the Health Professions, University of Pittsburgh, commented:

> The conduct and outcomes of this Project to date give real promise of a landmark study of lasting benefit to medical education. It is regrettable that medical educators are not more widely accepting of the worth of concerted effort in this area of improved teaching. Perhaps it will have to be largely at the experimental level for some time to come. More effective teaching in medical education would have tremendous long-range values to many beyond those involved directly in the process.

And the final comments in John Eberhart's field notes from April, 1957, read:

> In conclusion I want to say only that I think the experience of this first year has demonstrated the wisdom of [the Commonwealth Fund's] decision of eighteen months ago. This experiment in the improvement of medical school teaching hits directly at a central problem of medical education, and it has shown that knowledge and skill in this important area can benefit through the assistance of those for whom the study of education is a life work. In view of the traditional isolation of schools of education from other units of universities, this is an important demonstration. We may well find that in the years to come some of the young people who have participated in these programs will be among the leaders in medical education in the future.

Encouraged by this initial experience and the generally favorable judgment of program usefulness, the project staff approached the second year with considerably greater confidence. However, in light of that experience and those judgments, minor changes in the seminar program were agreed upon and two major extensions of the work were undertaken: acceleration of the educational research that had already been started, and initiation of a search for more economical means of introducing medical teachers to the science of education.

SECOND ROUND

Neither local nor national recruitment of participants was as easy in 1957-58 as it had been during the first year. At Buffalo, it proved impossible to win the involvement of any basic science group. The two departments that had participated during the first year were unable to release another individual for a second. Two other departments were in the unsettled state associated with a change in leadership, and the two remaining departments had been disinterested from the beginning. Among the clinical divisions, Pediatrics was eager to take part in the program; Medicine was willing to participate since a counterpart had already been identified; Obstetrics and Gynecology wanted to be represented once more even if a counterpart could not be found. Among the participants ultimately recruited (Table 3.1), the visiting faculty members were both older and more experienced than any of those in the first year. The entire group also proved to be more aloof in the beginning and less committed to the program after it got under way. In some part, at least, this may have been simply a reflection of the fact that these participants were more deeply involved in other things than their predecessors had been. For example, two local participants who were busy establishing research laboratories in their own hospitals were particularly sensitive to the importance of productivity in that sphere; a third was so committed to an increasingly demanding private practice that the time required for project work ultimately became burdensome. For one of the visitors, the opportunity to join a local research team for the year had been the major factor in his decision to participate in the project.

It was also true that these six individuals never succeeded in establishing a group identity. Part of this failure may have resulted from a change in seminar sequence. Participants in the first round had spent four hours each day, during the first week, in an intellectually demanding and emotionally intense analysis of the teaching-learning process. At the conclusion of this experience they had achieved a unity of purpose and a group strength that persisted throughout the year. During the second year, teaching-learning seminars were scheduled at weekly intervals. Whether for this reason or because of another unplanned change, the intensity of the experience was considerably reduced.

By late summer it had become clear that Cantor's illness was approaching a terminal phase. His forced withdrawal from the project was a great professional loss, and his death in October a great personal loss. At a considerable sacrifice Dr. Adelle Land, professor of education, stepped in at the last moment to fill the gap. She did an extraordinary job under very difficult circumstances, but there is no

TABLE 3.1. 1957-1958 Participants, Project in Medical Education

Participant	Department
Dr. Carmelo S. Armenia (University of Buffalo)	Instructor in Obstetrics and Gynecology
Dr. Albert G. Bickelman (University of Buffalo)	Research Fellow in Medicine
Dr. Mary O. Cruise (University of Louisville)	Visiting Assistant Professor of Pediatrics
Dr. Michael Matthews (University of Edinburgh)	Visiting Assistant Professor of Medicine
Dr. John R. Paul, Jr. (Medical College of South Carolina)	Visiting Associate Professor of Pediatrics
Dr. Clare Shumway (University of Buffalo)	Assistant Professor of Pediatrics

question that her low-key style and her lack of experience with medical education and physician teachers placed her at a great disadvantage. The seminar got off to an uneasy start from which it never completely recovered. Nonetheless, when the series ended, there was a general feeling among the participants that much of interest, and of use, had been dealt with.

The other seminar series were also found to be profitable. Yet none of the full-time participants was sure that the profit had been commensurate with the time invested — and that investment was, in the view of leaders, significantly less than had been made by the first group. Seminar leaders also agreed that they had experienced much greater difficulty during this second year in arousing and involving participants in both the seminars and the related activities. There appeared to be less personal commitment among them, less willingness to deal deeply with the problems posed by staff, and less initiative in defining problems for themselves. Although changes in attitude were clearly demonstrated through the systematic study that was conducted again by the Educational Research Center, these changes were neither as numerous nor as profound as those that occurred in the first group. Whether a third cadre would have responded more like the first or the second will never be known, for in the final years the program was substantially altered to meet some of the troublesome questions of practicality raised about an effort that required such a large investment of time, effort, and money, for a still questionable dividend.

CONCLUSION—FIRST PHASE

Edwin Rosinski had by now moved into a full-time post as research director for the project. In a final attempt to determine the impact of the program on those who had taken part in it, he conducted a one-year follow-up on twelve of the thirteen participants (he would have been pleased to follow the last member of the group as well, but a trip to Scotland was more than the project budget could sustain). In virtually every instance Rosinski was able to interview not only the participants themselves but also their department heads, a random sample of teaching colleagues and, in the case of visiting faculty, the medical school dean.

For ten of the twelve there was a consistent finding in self-reports and reports from associates that the project experience had resulted in discernible, significant, and persistent change in performance as a faculty member. Although the degree and kind of change varied among individuals, the direction was regularly toward application in practice of the educational principles that had been at the heart of the seminar and work/study experience. More rapid maturation, greater confidence, willingness to test alternatives and to accept differences, encouragement of students to discover what they needed rather than to absorb what they were told, a more questioning and less dogmatic approach to educational planning and implementation, and greater helpfulness to colleagues in finding new answers to old educational questions were among the most common changes reported. In only one instance was there a feeling that the program had produced a passion to convert others; in most the change was more often likened to a new spirit of inquiry about educational questions than to a posture of having found a final set of answers.

In general, the experience seemed to have been more valuable and to have produced a more significant impact on visiting participants than on those who were members of the Buffalo faculty. The visitors were able to participate in the professional activities of a vigorous medical school department without the attendant burden of heavy administrative, research, or teaching responsibilities, and to savor the delights of academic life without a sense of guilt about neglecting more mundane though necessary tasks. They had more freedom to explore the ideas being presented in the seminars as well as those being discovered in a new professional environment; they also had greater opportunity to read, to reflect, and to enjoy the accompanying excitement of planning how to use at home the things being learned while away. Upon return to the parent school, most of the visitors discovered that they were regarded as more expert resources in matters of departmental or school educational programs. Each was at the very least invited to present to one or more faculty groups the ideas that had emerged from the Buffalo experience and that had relevance to local problems. For most, the return also brought new opportunities for course organization or consideration of overall curricular problems.

The University of Buffalo participants, on the other hand, having gone nowhere and having been exposed only to an experience generated by local thoughts and visions (which were often controversial), frequently found themselves on the defensive. That at least five of them found something worthy of defense argues for the productivity of the experience. But there can be little question that the situation was more difficult for the Buffalo group not only because of the surrounding academic climate but also because they had more teaching, research, and administrative tasks during the study year than their visiting counterparts. Despite sincere efforts to relieve the Buffalo participants of a significant part of regular responsibilities, their continued presence and perceived availability made this arrangement work less well than had been planned.

For eleven of the thirteen participants, then, the experience appears to have been worthwhile. Whether it was worth the time invested we will never know. At the end of the work/study year most said it was not; twelve months later opinion was divided on this point, and at least some expressed regret that more time had not been devoted to specific areas of the seminar program. Did it make them better teachers? That would be very difficult to say. At least they ended with more information about the nature of learning, and about what teachers can do to influence this process as well as to assess its outcome. In most educational programs such a cognitive achievement is equated with success. However, project staff members were reluctant to accept this measure alone, for the real test is whether new knowledge is put to use in a manner that enriches a personal life or enhances the provision of a professional service. The available evidence suggests that this more stringent criterion may also have been met, at least for some of the participants.

Twenty years later each of the thirteen was asked to recall the year spent in the Project, and to reflect upon its worth. Nine responded with long and thoughtful comments. Without exception they still described the experience as one of considerable personal significance; some went so far as to say it had had a profound impact on their professional career development. Inevitably one wonders if these are merely the kind comments of old friends who have no wish to be other than generous. Yet as each gave specific illustrations of the influence of what had taken place two decades earlier, it was impossible to suppress a warm glow of satisfaction about the progress made in that provincial university toward breaking a barrier that had for so long separated two academic cultures.

PHASE TWO: A CHANGE IN DIRECTION

Initially, the project was designed as a five-year effort: a preparatory year followed by four one-year segments in which local and visiting faculty would engage in a work/study program. The three-year Commonwealth Fund grant was made with the understanding that a request for support of the final two years would be submitted if experience seemed to justify this extension. The project leaders and the advisory committee were now convinced that continuation was desirable, but they also recognized that a significant change in direction was essential if the program was to capitalize on the experience already gained. This conclusion was reflected in the ensuing application for program support during 1958-59 and for phase-out funds during a final year as the work became self-sustaining.

The new directions were four in number: (1) the development of greater opportunity for University of Buffalo Medical School faculty members to engage in more limited interaction with educational scientists; (2) the development of more economical methods of providing seminars and workshops in education for larger numbers of interested faculty from other schools; (3) the further elaboration of educational research efforts to match the educational development activities; and (4) the development of reference materials and workbooks that would be useful to others who might wish to embark upon similar teacher training programs.

Reaction of the Commonwealth Fund staff to this appeal is captured in a concluding paragraph of their review and comment:

In the report to the Board of November 1955 it was stated "The [Buffalo] program is based upon the obvious but sometimes overlooked fact that the heart of all education, medical or other, is learning. Therefore in order to cope successfully with the problems of medical education it is essential that the role of the teacher be both clarified and emphasized." This comment is as pertinent now as it was two and a half years ago. The Buffalo program, concentrating as it has on the function of the teacher in relation to student learning, has focused on a set of problems which in themselves are old but which have long needed new emphasis. The work of the project so far has been fruitful, and the activities proposed for the final year seem essential if the experience of this group is to be made available as widely as its merits suggest it should. In view of the Fund's continued interest in the improvement of medical education there seems ample justification for recommending [continued] support . . .

The board of directors responded with a terminal grant of $60,000, the amount requested for the final years.

BUFFALO FACULTY INVOLVEMENT

By design, the Project in Medical Education was at first limited to a small group of participants whose response to the study of educational principles could be carefully documented. Yet no one would deny an underlying hope that the program might have such apparent validity that it would stir up interest in the general medical faculty at the University of Buffalo as well as in other schools. What it did stir up at first was a considerable body of local skepticism and a moderate amount of hostility. There appeared to be a general disbelief that professional educators could make any significant contribution to the effectiveness of the medical school program, and a vague suspicion that the underlying purpose might really be to force the faculty into an educational pattern that project leaders had already agreed upon.

To counteract this feeling, invitational meetings held during the first year gave 125 medical school faculty members more detailed information about the program and an opportunity to question or challenge seminar leaders and participants. In addition, each of the visiting consultants took part in an open panel discussion on some educational topic of current interest or controversy. These methods, plus the informal questioning to which all those involved were regularly subjected, was reasonably successful in convincing the doubters that education might be a subject worthy of study, and that the project's purpose was to improve teaching, not to impose a new curriculum. Hostility perceptibly lessened; with increasing frequency faculty members asked how they might share this experience without devoting to it as much time as that demanded of regular participants.

To capitalize on this growing local interest, as well as to gain some impression of the relative usefulness of a less comprehensive program, each of the seminar series was opened during 1957-58 to a limited number of additional participants. The response was considerably greater than anticipated; three of the five topics were oversubscribed even though no special recruitment effort was made. However, these seminars were designed for those taking part in the full program; they were not planned as self-contained exercises and could not be expected to meet fully the interests of others. Thus in 1958-59 a modified set of seminar/workshops, aimed specifically at University of Buffalo educational problems and opportunities, was planned. On the basis of this experience, a design for subsequent years was to be developed.

For hope was now growing that this work might be institutionalized, that what had become a program of national interest would be fully reflected in the general medical education experience at Buffalo. It might have turned out that way if fate had not intervened. In February 1958, following a short illness, Stockton Kimball died. For those of us who regarded him as a close friend as well as a valued mentor, this was an irreplaceable loss. For the institution, his death precipitated a prolonged period of uncertain leadership. For the Project in Medical Education, it signaled the end of vigorous support in the highest faculty of medicine councils. Except for the personal sadness it produced, however, Kimball's death had no immediately discernible impact on the program; it was the subtle long-range effects that were ultimately so devastating.

MEETING A BROADER NEED

Providing access to ongoing seminars and planning short-term programs specifically for University of Buffalo School of Medicine faculty members addressed the local questions of practicality and economy but did not deal with the national issue. Most seminar leaders had now gained sufficient experience to be comfortable in considering more abbreviated offerings as an introduction to educational science. During the autumn of 1957 such a plan began to evolve; it took the form of an intensive two-week residential program that was tentatively scheduled for the early summer of 1958. Each of the general themes explored in the full-year program was to be included, but the separation into distinct categories was not as sharp. Content was culled, and only those elements that had proved to be most informative and provocative were included. Interrelationships among the several topics were emphasized both by the daily schedule and by the continuous presence of four leaders, who were joined by other resource persons during individual sessions. To ensure a totally absorbing experience, social events were integrated into the fabric of the program. These interludes provided temporary respite from intense intellectual involvement and also served as demonstrations of less formal learning experiences, as well as less familiar instructional methods. The final outline of activities is shown in Table 3.2.

It was generally agreed, however, that something more than solid substance might be required to attract attention. The University of Buffalo was not among the elite of American universities, and greater legitimization seemed necessary to assure a general acceptance of the premise that such an experience was worthwhile.

At each of the first three Teaching Institutes conducted in the early 1950s by the Association of American Medical Colleges (AAMC), there had been vigorous discussion of the proper methods of preparing medical teachers. Although opinions were expressed with great firmness and sometimes heat, they were rarely supported by data, by reference to the formal literature of educational research, or by the views of professionals drawn from that field. In his concluding comments about the first of these national faculty meetings, Julius Comroe wrote, "The Teaching Institute has spread the important truth that teaching as well as research is a proper concern of medical faculties and the design and examination of teaching methods should be both a challenge and stimulus to those engaged in medical education."[1] In this, as in subsequent Institutes, the idea of formal training in education for medical faculty members was at least brought forth, if not embraced. The University of Buffalo Summer Institute on Medical Teaching seemed to provide an opportunity for the AAMC to do something more than talk about this problem.

Thus it was that in January 1958, shortly before his death, Stockton Kimball extended to the Association of American Medical Colleges an invitation to join in sponsoring the two-week program. Ward Darley, executive director of the AAMC, took this invitation to the governing body with his endorsement, and in February replied to Dean Kimball that the Executive Council was "enthusiastic about the idea of joining the University of Buffalo in sponsorship of the forthcoming workshop on medical education." It was a critical breakthrough and set in motion a chain of events that had significant later effects on the Association and its membership. But most important at the moment was the AAMC agreement to sponsorship, a commitment that continued for four years.

An announcement of the Summer Institute was sent in April to the dean of each American and Canadian medical school, as well as to the chairmen of major basic science and clinical departments in these schools. It produced a flood of inquiries and applications, from which twenty-five participants representing twenty-one different schools were selected. The two-week experience in which they took part was extensively documented, and an evaluation was carried out using the now familiar log/diary and interview as well as a one-year follow-up by questionnaire. A detailed account of what happened appeared in the May 1959 issue of the *Journal of Medical Education*.[2] The outcome can be summarized simply: the Institute was an unqualified success.

Without exception, the participants agreed that the experience had been profitable. For many this outcome represented fulfillment of hope rather than expectation, because neither they nor their associates had had much confidence that professionals in education could offer anything of substantial usefulness to the teaching of medicine. Within three days this reservation had been dispelled; and by the end of two weeks there was general admiration for the educationists' professional skill and for their sophistication in dealing with problems of medical education. As one man put it, "the educators worked with us, not on us." Although there was some regret that the interprofessional team could not provide ready answers to all the immediate and long-range problems faced by medical teachers, there was also gratitude for the refreshing points of view,

TABLE 3.2. Schedule, First Summer Institute on Medical Teaching

	Sunday, June 15	Monday, June 16	Tuesday, June 17	Wednesday, June 18	Thursday, June 19	Friday, June 20
Morning		Introductory Presentations	Appraising Student Progress	Effective Use of Instructional Materials and Techniques	Problems of Learning	The Medical Student
		Coffee Discussion	Coffee Discussion	Coffee Discussion	Coffee Discussion	Coffee Discussion
Afternoon		Problems (Small Groups) Orientation to Campus	Group Discussion of Morning Topic Individual Problems— Review and Planning	Group Discussion of Morning Topic Individual Problems— Review and Planning	Group Discussion of Morning Topic Individual Problems— Review and Planning	Group Discussion Progress Reports
Evening	Social Gathering Faculty Club 8:30 p.m.				Dinner Faculty Club "Japanese Art and Music"	

	Sunday, June 22	Monday, June 23	Tuesday, June 24	Wednesday, June 25	Thursday, June 26	Friday, June 27
Morning		Overview of Higher Education	Techniques of Evaluation	Techniques and Materials of Instruction	Small Group Activities	Summation Criteria for Effective Instruction
		Coffee Discussion	Coffee Discussion	Coffee Discussion	Coffee Discussion	
Afternoon		Objectives of Medical Education	Small Groups	Individual Projects	Reporting Interviews	Evaluation
		Action Research	Achievement Tests			
			Clinical Performance Tests			
			Public Speaking			
			Graduate Education			
Evening		Dinner				
		Faculty Club				
		"Physician, Citizen and Courtier"				

backed by keen observation and sound reasoning, that they could provide.

When asked to cite specific gains derived from the Summer Institute experience, most participants referred to the new techniques of instruction and evaluation that had been brought to their attention, or to a new awareness of the strengths and weaknesses of more familiar methods of teaching and appraisal. Almost equally prominent were comments indicating modification of fundamental educational philosophy as a result of Institute explorations of the nature of learning and of the learner. This did not imply that participants left as "progressive" educators, whatever that ill-defined term might mean. Some of the more conservative or authoritarian were certainly convinced that moderation of their point of view was desirable, but one of the most liberal and permissive also concluded that some modification of this stance might benefit his students. Above all, participants recognized and accepted the fundamental importance of defining objectives before undertaking any educational program. How trite it seems now—but how fresh it seemed then.

Participants also noted that the organization, planning, and implementation of the Institute provided a daily illustration of the principles that were its substance. The leaders practiced what they preached. The housing arrangements, the conference facilities, the materials and methods of instruction, the planned breaks, the social events, and the very atmosphere reinforced the learning that was the goal of the conference. It was generally agreed that this learning objective could not have been achieved as easily, or as efficiently, had the same amount of seminar time been spread over six months or a year, had the program been offered to people living at home, or had individuals been housed in several residence halls. Because of constant proximity the participants worked as a group from the first day, and as a group they seemed to accomplish far more than a collection of individuals could possibly have done.

A question of central importance, probed in the final interview, was "Will this experience influence your teaching?" Without exception the response was affirmative. Some gave specific examples of contemplated course modifications or new methods of student appraisal that had been suggested during the Institute; others conveyed primarily a conviction that the experience could not fail to modify their teaching behavior even if the change involved no more than a deeper search for reasons why teaching was done in a particular way at a particular time, or for the motivations that produced unexpected student responses. At the very least, the participants expressed a heightened interest in education as a process.

When individuals were asked to describe weaknesses of the Institute program, there was no consistent or even dominant response. Almost everyone commented on the time span, but the comments ranged from pole to pole. One group felt the Institute had been too long, another wished it had been longer, while a third suggested that the time had been just about right. (The leaders felt that marked fatigue set in about the eighth day and that little progress was made during the final forty-eight hours.) There were several suggestions that a firmer hand would have allowed more rapid progress in the group discussions; others agreed, but added wistfully that the leaders had also shown there was more to teaching than covering the ground and that for the purposes of the Institute, their way may have been best. There was also some indication of disappointment that no opportunity to observe and analyze specific teaching sessions had been provided. Those who took part, though somewhat reluctantly, in a brief session on public speaking subsequently expressed regret that more time had not been given to the refinement of such basic teaching skills. Most of these observations were from single individuals or very small groups.

Two acts of the participants probably testify to the success of the Summer Institute far more than their words. At the concluding session, they proposed to reconvene in June 1959 in order to learn from each other how the experience had been translated into practice, and to consult once more with the staff. They also urged the extension of such opportunities to other groups in the future. But the most graphic testimony was a farewell dinner at a private club, given by participants for the leaders and their wives. The spirit, the table decorations, the gifts and poems, and particularly the skit that was a parody of the Institute provided all the data required to conclude that the two weeks had been a success.

This exhilarating experience was repeated in 1959, although the pressure for even greater economy led to truncation of the offering from two weeks to ten days. In 1960 it was further shortened to one week, the duration of the 1961 program as well. Over this four-year span 155 faculty members from 56 medical schools in the United States and Canada took part in the summer program. The immediate response of all participants and a one-year follow-up of those in the first three groups were summarized in a 1962 report to the medical education community, from which the following excerpt is taken:

> This report has brought together the personal appraisal of more than one hundred responsible faculty members who have described the ways in which they believe their behavior has in greater or lesser degree been modified by the seminar. Their general enthusiasm for, and their persistent belief in the usefulness of the experience is encouraging and lends greater strength to the hypothesis that the educational principles upon which the seminar is built are both practical and proper in the medical school.
>
> The initial purpose of the seminar was to encourage the individual medical faculty member to learn more about teaching and learning. We believe this purpose has usually been achieved but it is also clear that the influence of a single teacher upon the program of instruction to which a medical student is exposed will always be small. Participants have felt this limitation keenly as they returned to their own schools. In follow-up reports they have indicated in many ways the frustrations they experienced in attempting to convey to colleagues the content and the spirit of the seminar in a manner that would encourage a wider re-examination of institutional purpose and procedures. Their success has been limited and with the passage of time their discouragement has grown. A question repeatedly asked is whether exposure of a larger faculty sample of a single medical school to a common experience of this kind, and provision of continuing professional assistance in implementation of whatever intramural activity is agreed upon would have a greater impact on the total climate for learning within that institution.[3]

The question could not be answered then, but neither could it be ignored. It was an issue that influenced profoundly the later development of national and international programs alike.

ELABORATION OF EDUCATIONAL RESEARCH

The Project in Medical Education as a whole was regarded by its leaders as an applied research and development effort. However, two particular activities might fit the more common definition of fundamental and systematic research studies. Each was the outgrowth of an ingredient in the general program: modification of faculty attitudes toward education in medicine, and improvement of faculty performance in teaching. Both studies were integral parts of the whole, contributing new insight into the problems being explored in the project as well as providing new tools for assessment of what was being achieved.

Edwin Rosinski took major responsibility for the study of attitude change; Hilliard Jason carried similar responsibility for the study of teaching practices. Each had to begin by developing a method that would be technically acceptable and practically applicable. Only after this was done could the accumulation of data begin.

The use of interviews and log/diaries to document attitude changes in project participants has already been described. From this source Rosinski was able to extract roughly 1,500 specific attitudinal statements about the medical education process and setting. After repetitious and ambiguous items had been culled, the remaining 184 statements could be categorized in six broad areas, each of which included examples ranging from one polar extreme to the other. After further refinement and confirmation by independent judges, an attitude inventory of 120 statements distributed among the six areas (Table 3.3) was ready for preliminary trial. When the trial run revealed an acceptable level of statistical reliability and validity, the instrument was judged ready for more extensive use.

Documentation of change in individual teaching practices was included in the original project evaluation plan but was never accomplished. A major impediment to achieving this objective was the lack of an observational instrument that could be employed with confidence. Even though this component could not be included in the basic project evaluation, it remained a goal for the continuing effort, and a considerable investment was made in the development of a device that could serve this purpose.

Jason first created a comprehensive list of teaching characteristics, derived from a review of the literature and the suggestions of experienced teachers. These behavioral descriptions, when logically organized, fell naturally into seven subgroups. Each grouping was then reorganized into a continuum of possible teacher behaviors (Figure 3.2), with descriptive criteria for the polar extremes and two intermediate positions along an arbitrary twenty-unit scale (an illustration is given in Figure 3.3). After extensive review and refinement the instrument was used to train observers, in real and simulated

TABLE 3.3. Sample Category Items, Medical School Instructor Attitude Inventory

Category I	*Democratic:* "A close personal relationship between teacher and student improves the student's attitude toward his work."
	Autocratic: "The rigid use of authority in a classroom develops student respect for a teacher."
Category II	*Critical:* "The present medical school approach to education fails to teach the student to be a responsible individual."
	Complimentary: "Compared with other graduate schools, medical schools are doing as good or better a job of educating their students."
Category III	*Liberal:* "There is a need to look at what is going on in medical education in order to make changes that are needed."
	Traditional: "Department heads alone should be responsible for curriculum revision."
Category IV	*Appreciative:* "Medical school instructors should provide for individual student differences."
	Depreciative: "Medical students want to be spoon-fed in the classroom; that is, they want the cold, hard facts."
Category V	*Favorable full-time:* "The presence of full-time instructors has improved medical education."
	Unfavorable full-time: "Full-time clinical instructors do not possess any of the practical knowledge of medicine."
Category VI	*Favorable part-time:* "The part-time instructor plays an integral part in the medical school program."
	Unfavorable part-time: "Part-time teachers in medical schools have too many other responsibilities; teaching becomes incidental."

teaching settings, until an acceptable level of interrater reliability was achieved.

The major application of these devices took place in a study of teaching practices and faculty attitudes in seven American medical schools. The cooperation of these institutions, won through prolonged discussion and explanation, was both generous and understanding. Although the schools were selected with care to represent a cross section of settings for medical student education, the protection of anonymity led to identification only by the gross characteristics listed below:

1. An urban medical school not affiliated with a university.
2. An urban medical school, part of an Ivy League university.
3. An urban university medical school conducting a major experiment in medical education.

4. An urban university medical school, privately supported, with a predominantly full-time faculty.
5. An urban medical school, part of a sectarian university.
6. A state university medical school with a predominantly part-time or voluntary faculty.
7. A state university medical school with a predominantly full-time faculty.

Before the study ended, 380 teachers had completed a biographical information questionnaire and had been observed teaching in their regular classroom, laboratory, clinic, or ward by one or more members of the trained study team for a minimum of thirty minutes. One to seven months later, 247 of those observed completed the attitude inventory. With these data in hand, the investigators were able to compare and contrast the teaching practices and attitudes toward several elements of medical education between and among institutions, departments, age groups, professional degrees, class setting, and so forth.

Both the teaching practice and faculty attitude studies were descriptive, not judgmental. However, those who wanted to make judgments about the nature of instruction in representative American medical schools and the educational values held by a substantial sample of faculty members now had a systematically collected body of data on which to base those conclusions. They also had available two tested instruments for gathering further data if that seemed either necessary or desirable. In underscoring those points, Jason's report concluded with this observation:

Possibly the most significant feature of this study has been a demonstration that with an instrument such as the Medical Instruction Observation Record teaching can be examined with a fair degree of scientific precision. With such an approach the road is open for the study of the outcome of different instructional practices in terms of student performance. The findings of the present study do suggest that a sound knowledge of the relative effectiveness of different teaching approaches can have far reaching implications for our policies of academic appointment, curricular planning, class size and structure, and basic school organization. It is to be hoped that this vital question will be pursued with increasing vigor and sophistication.[4]

And Rosinski's report ended with these words:

Like many investigations this study has raised more questions than it has answered. One answer however seems clear. An in-

Scale 1 ATTITUDE TO DIFFERENCE	"A" End—Rejects questions that reflect poor understanding on the part of the student. Insults a student who disagrees with his own opinions. "T" End—Actively encourages group disagreement and discussion. Reacts to criticism with interest and understanding. Encourages individuals to express their points of view.
Scale 2 SENSITIVITY TO PHYSICAL SETTING	"A" End—No attention is paid to the physical comfort or needs of the group, in terms of: need for temperature change in the room, better view of the front, or a short recess. "T" End—Assures that everyone can hear all that is said, can see all that is written, and is comfortable. *Within the physical limitations of the room*, placement of both furniture and participants is utilized to maximum advantage.
Scale 3 ATTITUDE TO STUDENTS	"A" End—Active hostility to students is evident. Derogatory remarks are used, and an air of austere formality pervades the situation. "T" End—Acceptance and friendliness can be sensed at all times. Without necessarily being an accomplished humourist, the teacher sets a happy tone in his interaction with students. His interest in the students is readily felt.
Scale 4 USE OF INSTRUCTIONAL MATERIALS	"A" End—The material is poorly adapted to the situation, no introductory explanation is given, and no discussion accompanies or follows its presentation. It does not serve the purpose for which it was selected. "T" End—The material is well adapted to the apparent objectives of the session, its significance is made very clear, and the discussion during or following its use serves to highlight it.
Scale 5 REACTION TO STUDENTS' NEEDS	"A" End—The teacher forges ahead with the material he had prepared. He rejects student attempts at asking questions. He does not stop to question himself or the students as to whether his subject matter is actually geared to their interests and needs. "T" End—Repeatedly checks to insure that all students are grasping the material under discussion. Encourages questions when students begin to look puzzled, and detects students who are not participating.
Scale 6 USE OF TEACHING METHODS	"A" End—The method is poorly adapted to the size of the group, the teacher is not sufficiently familiar with it to have control of the situation, and it is not in keeping with the apparent objectives of the session. "T" End—The subject matter, group size, objectives, physical setting, and nature of the group, are all well served by the selected method. Appropriate materials are used to supplement the method; e.g., a motion picture is used to effectively illustrate points being presented. No ineptness in the use of the method can be detected.

FIGURE 3.2. Medical instruction observation record. Behavioral descriptions are used as extremes for six scales.

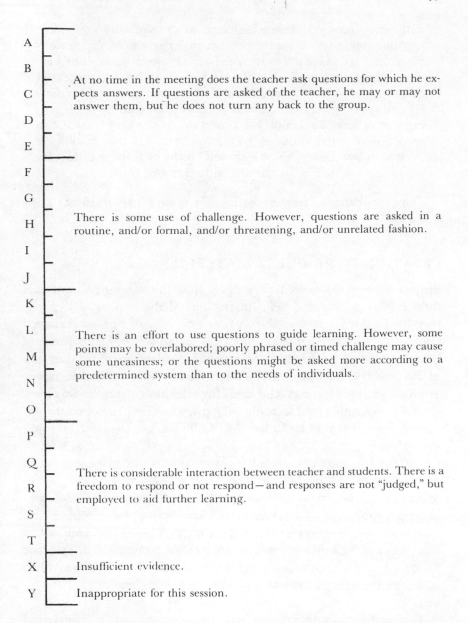

A
B
C At no time in the meeting does the teacher ask questions for which he expects answers. If questions are asked of the teacher, he may or may not answer them, but he does not turn any back to the group.
D
E
F
G
H There is some use of challenge. However, questions are asked in a routine, and/or formal, and/or threatening, and/or unrelated fashion.
I
J
K
L There is an effort to use questions to guide learning. However, some points may be overlabored; poorly phrased or timed challenge may cause some uneasiness; or the questions might be asked more according to a predetermined system than to the needs of individuals.
M
N
O
P
Q There is considerable interaction between teacher and students. There is a freedom to respond or not respond—and responses are not "judged," but employed to aid further learning.
R
S
T
X Insufficient evidence.
Y Inappropriate for this session.

FIGURE 3.3 Sample continuum, medical instruction observation record. Use of challenge (scale 7).

strument is now available which can, with reliability and validity, document in a more precise manner than impressions alone, the attitudes which may dictate faculty actions. The predictive usefulness of such a device has yet to be demonstrated but as a tool in the investigation of cause and effect of curricular change on modification in medical school climate for learning it may serve an important function. At the very least it can serve a descriptive purpose, to mirror an image that may have been seen but darkly. "Know thyself" is the beginning of faculty wisdom even as it is for the individual man.[5]

These conclusions seemed eminently reasonable in 1962. They still do.

CREATION OF RESOURCE MATERIALS

Project leaders discovered very early that the reference materials then available provided few illustrations of the educational problems medical teachers had to solve, or examples of how educational theory could be applied in the medical school setting. The personal experience of seminar leaders was generally adequate to fill that gap in the program itself, but if this work was to be extended to larger groups and other settings, the need for relevant references was inescapable. With this goal in mind, the proposal for project continuation through 1958-60 included a $15,000 budget item for creating such aids.

Initially the staff envisioned a set of workbooks to be produced under the general title *A Guide to Medical Teaching*. These introductory texts would be designed to provoke discussion about perplexing problems of curriculum and instruction, of teaching and learning, and of educational evaluation and research, and would also indicate the kinds of answers that could be extracted from the literature and experience of professional educators. Several films and tape recordings were also projected to supplement the written texts.

This ambitious undertaking was never completed in its original form. Roger Crane, director of the Commonwealth Fund Publication Division, wisely urged us to begin with a more conventional book. Even that proved to be a trying and time-consuming struggle for the seminar leaders who agreed to contribute to the volume. In the role of editor I also faced the not inconsiderable task of forging a consistent style and approach out of the individual formulations of five coauthors, while maximizing medical content and minimizing language that might be dismissed as educational jargon.

Preliminary drafts of several chapters, along with an outline of the remaining parts, went to Roger Crane in December 1958. His response was a welcome Christmas gift: Commonwealth Fund readers were all agreed that "the quality of both thinking and writing is gratifyingly high, and . . . that a very worthwhile publication will result." Encouraged, the authors now began to write in earnest, but the path to completion of their work was unexpectedly long and tortuous. Not until sixteen months later, in April 1959, was the completed manuscript finally submitted.

Editorial work by the Commonwealth Fund Publications Division staff began at once. We were particularly fortunate to have a highly competent, creative, and good-humored editor, Dorothy Obre, whose contributions were both significant and welcome. But all this work was only preliminary until the manuscript was accepted by the Harvard University Press, publisher of Commonwealth Fund books. The battle waged to win that acceptance vividly revealed the views that were then current about educational research and development in medicine.

The first hint that trouble was brewing came in an evaluation forwarded some six months later from a reader selected by the Press to make an independent assessment of the work's worth. In sum, this reviewer expressed serious doubt about whether the manuscript, at least as it had been submitted, was worthy of publication. While acknowledging that the authors were clearly expert in the field of general education, the reader judged their knowledge of medical education to be superficial, their definition of the central issues in that field unsophisticated, and their proposed solutions naive. The reviewer was also annoyed by what he (she) perceived as an overall tone of complaint about limited interest among seemingly self-satisfied medical faculty members in learning more about sound educational principles, and especially in learning them from those qualified in the discipline of education. The most positive suggestion was that the book might usefully be rewritten as a general education text, using the data drawn from medical education simply for illustration, and thus avoiding a flavor sensed in the original version that the volume was regarded by the writers as equivalent to another Flexner report.

I was stunned by the attack, having naively concluded that we had already weathered this kind of storm. But Roger Crane, his support unshaken, was more realistic. His guidance now was as helpful as it had been in the past, and would prove to be again in the future. He began with a gentle reminder that the number of medical educators who believed educationists could be useful to them was still small, and the reviewer was clearly not among them. Crane then suggested a dispassionate response, drawing upon the experience we had by now accumulated, and avoiding the heated reply that such a review might easily provoke. He also assured us that the manuscript had been sent to two additional readers who seemed more likely to belong to the now growing group who might agree that medical educators could still learn something about education from disciplines other than their own.

During the next week I composed what seemed like an eloquent response. Nearly twenty years later, rereading it still stirs the blood. However, following the good advice that had been given, passion was tempered by reason, and only a few major points were made. The first was directed at documenting the authors' qualifications in medicine and in education (it was difficult to resist the jibe that the educationists among them had spent more time studying medical schooling than more than a few medical faculty members had ever spent studying education). Secondly, attention was drawn to the conclusion reached by nearly 100 medical teachers from 48 medical schools who had by then participated in summer programs that the general principles and suggested practices set forth in the book were indeed useful in fact, not in theory alone.

When the additional reviews came in two months later, one reader recommended publication, but only with significant modification of content; the second was much more positive, but qualified his favorable comments with an unexpected observation that he had initially failed to grasp the intent of the volume, and only later realized that it was designed to teach teachers something about teaching and learning, not to report new data or studies about medical education. In the light of all these comments we came to the conclusion, which was shared by Roger Crane, that some of the suggestions made by the reviewers had merit, but that the major alterations they proposed would weaken rather than strengthen the work. These views were conveyed to the editor, and through him to the Board of Syndics. After considering the arguments on both sides the Board members agreed, at their December 1960 meeting, to accept the manuscript for publication with the proviso that the recommendations made by the readers would be carefully considered by the authors, after which final text changes would be negotiated with the science editor of the Press. The most important modification upon which consensus was quickly reached was the insertion of a completely rewritten preface, one that would deal with some of the questions and challenges raised by the reviewers and would also clarify the intent of the book. The revised manuscript went back to the Press early in February. It was promptly accepted by the editor, and was finally published on June 14, 1961.[6] During the next thirteen years the English language edition went through three printings; Spanish and Portuguese versions appeared in the middle 1960s, and a Japanese translation was published in 1978, four years after the Harvard University Press edition went out of print. I have often wondered if the first reader ever had second thoughts about his comments, particularly if he happened to see a review in the Journal of the American Medical Association that read in part:

> The authors adequately discredit the adage that "teachers are born, not made" . . . Indeed *Teaching and Learning in Medical School* is such a direct attack on insularly held cherished beliefs and practices rampant in our medical schools, that one wonders if even so called unbiased and open-minded scientists can bring themselves to digest its content . . . It could well modify teaching attitudes and techniques much as Flexner's report modified the medical school curriculum. With such potential it should be required reading for all who profess to teach medicine.[7]

DECLINE AND FALL

Ironically, by the time *Teaching and Learning in Medical School* was published the program that had spawned it was moribund, if not dead. The overt manifestations of impending disintegration appeared at the end of the 1958-59 academic year, when three major figures in the project moved on to pursue other opportunities in more promising settings, but the covert manifestations of waning vigor began to be felt following Stockton Kimball's death one year earlier. None of the deans who succeeded Kimball (and there were three during the period from 1957 to 1960) took the same personal interest in the program or gave it the same personal support as he had. Their priorities were different, or at least they were less willing to buck the tide that periodically ran against the concepts embodied in the Project in Medical Education.

The final year of external funding (1959-60) had been planned as a period of transition to continued internal support. It was a year spent trying to identify more precisely what the University of Buffalo could and would do on its own. With my departure in September 1959, responsibility for project direction was given to two of the young faculty members who had been participants in the first-year program: Donald Becker, a surgeon, and Murray Blair, a pharmacologist who had recently returned from Tufts to become a permanent faculty member at Buffalo. Becker and Blair later expressed a feeling that their lack of administrative experience probably contributed to some of the problems encountered during the final year. However, an observer from afar can only be impressed that they were able to sustain as much momentum as they did.

The program pattern that emerged during 1959-60 was not unlike that which Edward Bridge had initiated nearly ten years earlier: a weekly seminar on medical education for interested faculty members, with resource persons drawn from other university divisions and particularly from among those who had been earlier contributors to the project. The new leaders discovered again, however, that educationists who were unfamiliar with the realities of medical education were generally disdained by medical teachers, no matter how respected those experts might be in their own field.

The new project directors also tried to capitalize on the Summer Institute experience but were forced by local circumstances to settle for a two-day retreat. Nonetheless, this occasion provided an unusual opportunity for communication among the sixty University of Buffalo School of Medicine faculty members who attended. It was, however, a very different experience from the carefully orchestrated program of prior years when the focus had been on educational process rather than on local issues.

At the end of the 1959-60 academic year Blair left the University of Buffalo, and Becker was now alone in the leadership role. While deeply committed to the project, he was also a practicing surgeon whose time for guiding and administering the program was very limited. Becker felt the loss of Murray Blair for another reason as well: it broke the symbol of an integrated effort by basic and clinical scientists together. During 1960-61 the continuing seminar involved primarily clinicians and used the talents of the most experienced resource persons from education. But the pace was clearly slower, and the spirit of adventure was gone.

In February 1961, Becker's summary account of the project reached the Commonwealth Fund. The final paragraph reflects his personal judgment of what the work had meant to the University of Buffalo:

> Insofar as a major break-through is concerned, the golden point, in retrospect, was probably 1956-57, when decisive action and official sanction of the medical administration would probably have spelled the difference between success and failure of the program at a level high enough to have had significant repercussions on the curriculum and faculty. The fact that the administration has been in an unstable position with two Deans and an Acting Dean within this period is one of the major factors of this hesitant position. As a result the general consensus appeared to be that the Project in Medical Education was an interesting investigation, more tolerated than sponsored by the administration. In that the program never really got off the ground from this standpoint it must be considered a failure. It will require a number of years for the junior faculty members who participated in the program to reach administrative heights before it will be finally determined whether or not the piecemeal gains do add up to final success.

A covering letter from the acting dean of the School of Medicine may appear to confirm this view. He reported an unexpended balance of $20,007.81 from the final grant, which he was returning to the Fund.

Attached to the Commonwealth Fund file copies of those last documents is a handwritten note by John Eberhart: "A rather touching and somewhat sad final report on a noble experiment at Buffalo, a school with its troubles. It didn't set the Buffalo medical school on fire but that now appears not to have been very combustible. It did have some good wider influences."

It is to those influences that we now turn.

INITIAL COLONIZATION

4

Although they would probably deny having had any aspiration to the role of proselytizers, the leaders of the Project in Medical Education were from the beginning committed to the idea of program outreach. At the very least they expected that the half of each participant group returning to parent institutions would share with colleagues the ideas they had acquired and the experience they had gained in Buffalo. A steady flow of interested visitors through the project office, even during the first year, supported a belief that others might also profit from what we were learning about how teachers could more effectively use themselves to further the educational enterprise in medical schools. Such belief was given additional impetus when an invitation came to describe the Buffalo experience at the June 1957 annual meeting of the N.I.H. Cardiovascular Teaching Grant Coordinators. This first public presentation was particularly challenging because it was to be paired on the program with the well-established and widely admired Western Reserve experiment.

The acknowledgment of more general utility, not to mention acceptability, of educational science in the medical school was further fostered when two of the project staff were asked to serve as major resource persons at the first University of Michigan School of Medicine Teaching Institute in 1958. But it was the enthusiastic response of participants in the first Summer Institute that stimulated serious thought among project leaders and the advisory committee about developing a systematic plan for colonization.

These thoughts finally crystallized in a new proposal, submitted to the Commonwealth Fund in December 1958, which was called "A

Study to Determine the Impact of an Educational Consultant on a Medical School." The plan included four stages:

1. *Preparation.* Experience had now demonstrated convincingly that a professional educator, to be successful in the field of medicine, first needed some general orientation to the content, the language, the climate, the values, the substance of that world. An intensive preparatory period, not unlike that through which project seminar leaders had passed, would be required before consultants took up residence in the five projected study schools.

2. *Matching.* In order to provide maximal opportunity for success, such a consultant must be not only well qualified for the role but also acceptable to the school. Although preliminary sounding had suggested the existence of a potentially interested and qualified pool of personnel and institutions, it was necessary to gain from five individuals and five schools a firm commitment to one another for the two- to three-year study period that was proposed.

3. *Implementation.* Because the interests and needs of each study school would be different, it was impossible to predict accurately the specific services that each consultant would provide. They might serve school-wide educational committees, departmental groups struggling with educational problems, or individual faculty members trying to improve pedagogic skills; they might offer seminars or workshops on general educational issues or specific educational problems; they might identify other professional or technical resources in education that would be of use to the school or serve as a liaison with resources already present but unused in the institution. In the face of such varied possibilities, continuing assistance from the core group in Buffalo was also built into the program.

4. *Assessment.* In addition to a personal log of activities carried out during the two- to three-year study period, each consultant, along with a sample of administrative personnel, instructional staff, and students, would be asked at some point to judge both the impact of the consultation and its worth. The most significant piece of positive evidence would be continuation of the consultant's appointment after external subsidy was terminated.

As project staff members worked together on developing the proposal, mounting enthusiasm for what seemed to be the natural extension of a successful demonstration program could be felt throughout the Buffalo team. With the prospect of major project activities coming to an end in August 1959, the most involved of the professional educators found themselves even more committed to medical education than they had realized: Rosinski was attracted by the possibility of serving as one of the five proposed consultants; Abrahamson was prepared to undertake the systematic assessment of consultant impact; Harnack was ready to serve as field supervisor of the consultants. Enthusiasm was evident outside Buffalo as well. Among the twelve medical schools to which informal inquiries were sent, ten indicated that they would welcome the opportunity to have an educational consultant-in-residence. All that was now needed was the money to make it possible.

That item the Commonwealth Fund finally decided it was not prepared to provide. Despite a generally sympathetic reception of the proposal, the Fund staff reluctantly concluded in January 1959 that they could not then justify support for a program of this magnitude (the projected budget was slightly more than $360,000). They were, however, prepared to continue discussion of possible alternatives, and that discussion, with Lester Evans and Charles Warren, took place in Chicago during the February Congress on Medical Education. In the course of four hours it was agreed that the most feasible means for determining whether the idea had merit was to place such a consultant in one school and see what happened. It took only a few minutes to identify the school that seemed best prepared for such an experience. Of all the institutional leaders who had expressed interest, Dean William Maloney at the Medical College of Virginia was most eager to move promptly. As a result of prior encounters, he and Rosinski were both convinced that the match between them would be a good one. This feeling was captured in Warren's field notes of further exchanges among the interested individuals that took place over the next two days:

> At present there is [at the Medical College of Virginia] a committee on education composed of forty members of the faculty, and a planning committee of six members. These groups meet approximately weekly to review the educational program at Virginia and to make plans for changes. Maloney is convinced that an educator like Rosinski would serve a most useful function if appointed as consultant to the committee on education. He would have a focus of his activities here, and would be available for consultation by the committee as a whole, individual members of the committee, and individual members of the faculty . . .

During the past year Rosinski has been to Richmond twice . . . During these visits he was accepted by the faculty without the slightest prejudice, and Maloney feels that he would work well with this group . . . Dean Maloney also feels strongly that the work of such an educational consultant should be approached in a framework of research and evaluation . . .

We did not have time to discuss in detail the relevance of research to this experimental use of an educational consultant, but I found that I personally was much readier to accept such an approach when it was outlined with respect to a specific medical school and a specific educator, than when the matter is dealt with in generalities.

On the basis of his discussion this seemed to me very close to an ideal setting for the kind of experiment we were discussing . . . Since Rosinski has been involved in the activities of the Buffalo program almost from the beginning he would be a good person to lead off such an effort.

Three weeks later Maloney submitted a formal request to the Commonwealth Fund for financial assistance that would allow the addition of an educational consultant-in-residence to the Medical College of Virginia staff. In April the site visit by Warren and Eberhart produced a positive recommendation: "This proposal is a natural for the school . . . stemming as it does from their exposure to the Buffalo program." In May the Commonwealth Fund board of directors approved the grant, and in July Edwin Rosinski moved to Richmond as a lecturer in medical education and a consultant to the Committee on Medical Education. The first colony had been established.

It was a thriving enterprise for seven years, one that demonstrated not merely the viability of a concept, but also the concrete contributions that could be made by a professional educator-in-residence to the educational program of a medical school. This conclusion was supported most persuasively when in 1961 the College established a formal Office of Research in Medical Education, and one year later, upon termination of the Commonwealth Fund grant, assumed financial responsibility for this work.

Undoubtedly the unremitting support of Dean Maloney was a critical element in gaining this degree of acceptance, but the rapidity with which it was accomplished is a tribute to Rosinski's skill in meeting the challenges and exploiting the opportunities he encountered. Reflecting on how it all occurred, he recently attributed this success in no small measure to ". . . a lesson I learned from Bob Harnack as a graduate student, namely, get as many people involved in what you are doing as possible. Right from the start that lesson was my credo. By the time I left MCV almost 65% of the faculty was involved in (or were participating in) some activity related to improving the quality of the educational program. The chairman of one of my key committees, a professor in the basic sciences, said it best: 'When you arrived, Rosinski, I assumed a conspiracy was afoot. There isn't! Anything I am involved in cannot be a conspiracy.' " Rosinski managed to achieve this involvement through many tactics, but the basic strategy was that of using every possible opportunity to convince the faculty that he was there to help them do better what they wanted to do, not to tell them what they should be doing. The message was communicated as often in a fishing boat as in a seminar room. Yet even the soft sell of unfamiliar things inevitably engenders some anxiety. As one of the leaders later put it: "He scared the faculty to death by asking them what their objectives were, and suggesting that we study our program for content, objectives, etc."

Even when they were frightening, however, such suggestions often led to fruitful work. Before long virtually all departments of the school were, with Rosinski's help, developing explicit teaching objectives and taking part in an institution-wide effort to document who was teaching what, where, and when. The subject matter cataloging system,[1] the centerpiece of this effort, was not only a notable achievement in itself but also provided the mechanism that greatly facilitated development of a new curriculum when this became a high educational priority at MCV.

Although he believed that increased faculty familiarity with a wider range of educational principles was best achieved through participation in such work, the consultant-in-residence also kept faculty members informed about more general issues and techniques through distribution of reprints, publication of a newsletter, and organization of faculty retreats at which educational as well as administrative topics were discussed. He worked with the committee on instructional methods to improve teaching, with the committee on examinations to review testing and grading practices, with individual faculty members who asked for help in improving their teaching skills, and with all those who sought assistance in improving the dynamics and productivity of their working groups.

In short, Rosinski was engaged in all the kinds of professional services that had been envisioned for a consultant-in-residence in the original study proposal. In addition, he continued with his educational research. The interest aroused by the medical faculty attitude inventory led him to develop a student attitude inventory, using very similar methodology. And when a completely new curriculum was finally mounted in 1963, he was instrumental in developing and carrying out a long-term evaluation that has only recently been completed.

Despite this remarkable accomplishment, the road was not always smooth. A bitter town-gown battle erupted in the mid-1960s, purportedly over the values embodied in the new curriculum to which Rosinski had made such a significant contribution. Although the ruckus did not directly affect Rosinski's work, it probably contributed to the downfall of Dean Maloney, who had been the major sponsor and a continuing supporter of the educational research and develoment effort. The work itself was draining, both emotionally and intellectually, for the budget had never been large enough to provide an adequate professional staff for the number of projects in which the Office of Research in Medical Education was engaged. In addition to coping with this internal struggle, Rosinski was also broadening his horizons. As a Rockefeller Foundation consultant and an advisor to the U.S. Agency for International Development, he was challenged particularly by the problems associated with the education of other health workers, especially that relatively new category known as a physician's assistant.

By 1966 he needed a respite, if not a permanent change of responsibility. Such an opportunity appeared when Phillip Lee, assistant secretary for health and scientific affairs in the Department of Health, Education, and Welfare, invited Rosinski to become his deputy. Although the departure from the Medical College of Virginia was billed as a temporary leave of absence, he never returned to the post that had been occupied with such distinction for seven years.

Nor was he replaced. Although several candidates were interviewed, none was appointed. When asked ten years later why the position had not been filled, Kinloch Nelson, who had been dean at the time, said, "The only reasons I know why we did not replace Ed promptly after 1967 are on the one hand, funds were low, and on the other, we could not find a suitable person." However, during 1967-68 twelve other medical schools managed to find qualified directors of new educational research and development offices, and one would have thought that an institution with MCV's record could have attracted the best of the growing pool of trained candidates. Despite the disarming words, it is difficult to avoid an impression that the leadership commitment was not there.

And so the first colony became little more than a ghost town, filled with memories and promise. It was another somewhat sad ending to a tale that was filled with excitement and achievement. But it proved to be not really an ending, merely the beginning of a period of dormancy. The work was rejuvenated in 1972 through a newly established Educational Planning and Development Program that now serves the entire Virginia Commonwealth University Health Science Center, of which the Medical College of Virginia is a part. Thus the old settlement has taken on new life.

By then, however, Rosinski had himself moved on, first to establish an educational research program at the new University of Connecticut Medical School, then to a vice chancellorship at the University of California Medical Center in San Francisco, and later to the directorship of the Office of Education there. From that site his personal contributions to medical education research and development are continuing.

The second colony was little more than a temporary outpost, nor was it planned to be anything beyond that. Nonetheless, it represents a significant part of the evolutionary tale and thus deserves recounting.

The beachhead was established by Stephen Abrahamson, who by 1959 had become so caught up in the world of medical education (and so widely recognized for his contributions) that he was reluctant to abandon the challenges this new field represented. It was a great disappointment to him when our proposal to study the impact of professional educators-in-residence on selected medical schools was not funded, since he had looked upon this study as the kind of continuing opportunity that would have brought great personal as well as professional satisfaction. Now some new course had to be found if he were not to become fully immersed once more in the University of Buffalo School of Education (a return to the fold that Dean Fisk would have welcomed).

In his growing acquaintance with medical educators, Abrahamson had encountered many individuals with whom he had established an almost instant sense of compatability. One of these was Lyman Stowe, associate dean of the Stanford University Medical School, which had recently moved from San Francisco to the Palo Alto campus and was engaged in a major curriculum revision. Stowe wanted desperately to have the help of a real professional in education and had convinced Dean Robert Alway that in Abrahamson he had found the man. Alway agreed to find the money to bring this expert to Stanford for a year if he could be induced to come.

It was not an easy decision for Abrahamson. The move meant a more complete separation from his own discipline and professional colleagues than he had contemplated, but it did provide an opportunity to test whether he could make the career shift comfortably and successfully. The offer was finally accepted with some apprehension, but with a great sense of challenge (an opportunity to escape the Buffalo snows for a year was not unappealing either).

In 1959, the Stanford University campus was an exciting place for an adventurer embarking on the sea of medical education. It was a time of change in institutional values and aspirations as the clinical disciplines, which had for so long existed separately in San Francisco, were brought into the mainstream of university life in Palo Alto. This fresh spirit in education, research, and patient care was superbly symbolized by the magnificent new medical school/hospital structure in which Edward Durell Stone captured again the openness and beauty that characterized the American Embassy building he had created in New Delhi.

The new medical curriculum, which students were to embark upon for the first time that September, had been shaped in part by the Western Reserve model but broke even further from established tradition and current fashion. At a time when most schools were talking about reducing the years of medical education, Stanford boldly extended the program from four years to five. But the extension in time was accomplished by consolidation and diversification rather than expansion in uniform and planned instruction for all students. The new course of study was designed to obliterate the sharp interface between premedical and medical education, to reduce the core content for all students while increasing individualized study opportunities for each, and to shift the educational focus from fostering simple acquisition of facts to developing critical problem-solving skills. The most significant new elements in program design included: (1) providing the equivalent of one academic

year of "university time," spread over the first three years of instruction, during which those few students admitted without a baccalaureate could complete requirements for that degree, while others
could enroll in any general university courses they found appealing;
(2) integrating the teaching of all basic sciences, using multidisciplinary laboratory experience as a major instructional device; (3)
steadily increasing the exposure to clinical medicine over the first
three years, culminating in an introduction to the historical and
philosophical aspects of medicine; (4) organizing required clinical
work as interdepartmental offerings during the final two years; and
(5) ensuring a significant amount of elective time throughout the
curriculum.

Appealing as this general outline seemed, it had been developed
by individuals trained in the biomedical disciplines—faculty members who were experienced in medical teaching but were generally
unfamiliar with educational science. Thus it was understandable
that the details of planning for implementation might not match
the elegance of conceptual design. Under these circumstances the
challenge that faced an educational consultant (also titled Visiting
Professor of Education) was not insignificant. How to meet that
challenge was rather less clear. Unlike Rosinski, who was an integral
part of the faculty structure at the Medical College of Virginia,
Abrahamson was a visitor at Stanford; he had no formal assignment
or responsibility and no established place in the academic hierarchy
of the school. The strategy and tactics he finally adopted were later
described in this way:

> In our earlier discussions, Dr. Stowe and I saw a three-fold
> approach . . . (1) We thought that a series of seminars might be
> arranged for interested faculty members to attend. In those
> seminars general principles of measurement and evaluation
> would be covered and the specific problems of participants in
> the seminars would be studied by the seminar group. (2) Sub-
> ject committees of the faculty would be encouraged to solicit
> my assistance as those committees engaged in discussions per-
> taining to evaluation. (3) Individual faculty members would be
> encouraged to consult with me as they became faced with prob-
> lems in appraisal and evaluation.
>
> The seminar approach was deemed the most important be-
> cause it seemed to offer the greatest opportunity for the faculty
> of the medical school to become aware of my existence and my
> potential contribution. The third approach, that of awaiting

individual faculty member requests, was deemed the least important since there was so much left to chance.

It was in the area of the second approach that I was able to make my contribution to the faculty of the School of Medicine. In fact, the early acceptance of my potential contribution by the faculty eliminated the anticipated need for the seminar sessions. During the first several weeks of my stay here, I became so involved in the workings of several subject committees on which were serving most of the faculty members who had expressed interest in the seminars, that Dr. Stowe and I postponed indefinitely the beginning of any seminar session. All that I might have been able to accomplish in the seminar sessions was much more easily and much more meaningfully covered as I met with these subject committees. In those situations the same material was explored and a deeper understanding of the principles of education was achieved through the group attempt to solve real and specific problems . . .

These real and specific problems fell into two broad areas: (1) further refinement of objectives; and (2) development of student assessment procedures.

In these days when references to Mager and Gronlund flow so easily from the tongues of medical curriculum planners, and full volumes of instructional objectives cast in behavioral terms guide student learning and faculty teaching in many medical schools, it may be difficult to picture a time when things were not this way. But that time was only a score of years ago. It may be understandable, then, that when an educational consultant appeared on the scene of a new medical school in 1959, his initial response to faculty requests that he tell them how to teach or how to evaluate students would take the form of a simple and logical question: "What do you expect them to learn?" Getting an answer, however, was much more difficult and time-consuming, as Abrahamson discovered again and again in working with staff members responsible for the outpatient program, the basic clerkship, the child health program, and introduction to clinical medicine. The task was not so much that of getting medical teachers to use the technical language of education in specifying their objectives as getting them to clarify and make explicit what the objectives really were. For example, Abrahamson recalled that with one group, "one solid hour was spent on whether a rectal examination was properly to be expected of all medical students as part of the routine physical examination [of an adult] . . .

Considerable time was spent attempting to define the criteria which differentiate outpatient medical practice from inpatient." But the documents that resulted from these efforts with responsible program groups, work that extended over the full year of his consultation, were both revealing to the faculty participants and impressive to external reviewers.

The greatest progress, however, was made in the evaluation of student performance. Working from course objectives, now more precisely defined, faculty members were able to develop with Abrahamson's help a remarkable set of observational rating scales for the outpatient program, the child health program, and the basic clerkship. His carefully designed study of essay examination reliability provided a model for the best construction and use of this evaluation instrument, even as it demonstrated the gross and meager nature of information on student performance that is provided by even the most careful employment of this assessment method. On another tack, by dispassionately documenting what took place in a departmental student grading session Abrahamson was able to illustrate how little sound information may be exchanged in such deliberations, and to what extent opinion or inference based on limited sampling may influence those decisions. (For example, in one instance a student was described initially as "basically interested in the work; he just doesn't have the intelligence," whereas moments later a second observer commented, "he has the intelligence, but he is obviously not interested," while other members of the faculty nodded agreeably at both judgments.) Finally, Abrahamson had an opportunity to introduce into Stanford's individualized educational program the idea that peer ratings of student performance might provide another important piece of data from which to determine whether the objectives of this unique approach were being achieved.

It will not have escaped the perceptive reader that all this work was done with clinical groups. If one can detect any expression of disappointment in Abrahamson's account of the year as consultant-in-residence, it was that his only opportunity to work with the basic sciences was in a single meeting of the Committee on Cell Structure and Function, during which members were discussing the preparation of an examination. In a medical school that gave such importance to attitudinal learning and in the face of the difficulty of modifying attitudes without institution-wide reinforcement through consistency in instructional climate and evaluation procedures, it would have seemed particularly advantageous for the school to have exploited the potential contribution of a professional educator in the basic sciences as well as in the clinical programs. The fact that it did not may in part reflect a conflict in values with which Stanford was then struggling.

For the medical school was clearly trying to establish a new image, not only in its educational philosophy but also in its research productivity and its service arrangements. The move from San Francisco to Palo Alto was more than geographic: it also represented a major shift in institutional orientation, a shift that was significantly influenced by a new cast of faculty characters who identified more closely with the things academicians prize than with those practitioners value. The most turbulent time was still ahead, but the rumblings were already apparent. In the face of these brewing conflicts, the contribution made by an educational consultant in the course of a single academic year is even more impressive.

If Lyman Stowe had had his way, the work would not have ended then and Abrahamson would not have returned to Buffalo. But the leadership at Stanford had other priorities, which slowly submerged much of what had been accomplished during this productive interlude. Virtually no institutional residue of Abrahamson's work persisted, and Stanford never went on to establish a formal medical education research and development group. However, through two individuals at least, the work produced significant repercussions elsewhere. When Stowe became dean of the newly established medical school at the University of Connecticut, he took with him many of the ideas and attitudes he had acquired during that year. An even more important transplantation occurred when Andrew Hunt, a pediatrician and major colleague in this year-long consultation at Stanford, became founding dean of the Michigan State University School of Human Medicine. One of Hunt's first actions was to establish an Office of Medical Education Research and Development, which became a centerpiece for educational planning, program implementation, and student evaluation in that new program.

Thus at Stanford a second colony was born, flourished briefly, and then vanished leaving scarcely a trace. But the experience did influence the colonizer: Abrahamson returned to Buffalo for only two years, then moved west once more to establish at the University of Southern California what has now become one of the three most prominent medical education units in the United States.

In the meantime, a third Buffalo outpost took shape on the medical center campus of the University of Illinois in Chicago.

It is probably fair to say that the ground at the University of Illinois College of Medicine had been more thoroughly prepared to receive an educational research and development implant that at either the Medical College of Virginia or Stanford. Dean Granville Bennett, a pathologist turned administrator, had given substantial encouragement during the late fifties to an expanding group of young faculty members who were committed not only to improvement of the institutional program of medical education, but also to achieving that goal through the process of scholarly study, not by zeal alone. For example, Dr. Nicholas Cotsonas had undertaken a systematic analysis of the student-instructor interaction in the general medical clinics; Dr. Max Samter had initiated an extensive observational analysis of clinical lectures; Dr. George Jackson, and others on the admissions committee, had conducted a revealing investigation of group interviews in the selection process; and Dr. Adrian Ostfeld had launched an impressive longitudinal study to determine how graduates were influenced in their practice by the education experienced in the school and the forces encountered after graduation.

Encouraged by these individual and group efforts, which had already produced local changes in curriculum and instruction, and anticipating a growing pressure upon tax-supported institutions to increase their size, Bennett raised with faculty the question of whether Illinois, one of the nation's largest medical schools, might be an appropriate site for educational experimentation of the kind that had up to then been carried out primarily by small, privately supported schools. Sensing an affirmative response, he turned, as had so many others, to the Commonwealth Fund as a potential source of financial assistance for such an effort.

The conversations that were initiated with the foundation in 1958 led Lester Evans to spend a week in May on the Medical Center and Urbana/Champaign campuses of the University. His long memorandum describing the visit is revealing in many ways; particularly significant were these excerpts:

> I am not yet able to understand fully why this school should have gotten such a good start in studies of medical education . . . but the fact remains that very few schools have done as wide a range of work as this . . .
>
> Possibly the greatest single factor is in the quality of the faculty. They are faced with an enormous educational problem and are desirous of doing the best possible job as teachers . . .

The nearest brief characterization I can give of the faculty group I saw and the enthusiasm with which they entered in the discussion of problems under consideration is that they are as much like the Western Reserve faculty of the early days of their educational program as any group I have seen . . .

Evans went on to describe the unusual setting of the University of Illinois Health Professions Colleges as the "spiritual center" of a 300-acre West Side Medical Center that also included two other medical schools, the Cook County Hospital, the Presbyterian-St. Luke's Hospital, and the West Side Veterans Administration Hospital, as well as the University's Research and Educational Hospitals and a spate of specialized municipal and state health service organizations. He noted the unusual resources that were available to the medical school through other University divisions in Chicago and Urbana/Champaign. Evans was particularly impressed by the commitment of campus and general university administrators to collaborative efforts that would contribute to the strength of all divisions. And finally, he noted the generous incremental budget that lent stability to the university enterprise. In fact, his only real concern appeared to be the size (not the quality) of the student body. Yet even this struck him as opportune, since it represented an almost inevitable aspect of the future to which most medical schools would need to adapt.

The optimism that appeared in Evans' notes must have been conveyed in his words to the dean, for six weeks later a formal proposal requesting support for the "Study and Evaluation of Medical Education at the University of Illinois College of Medicine" was received by the Commonwealth Fund. Unlike the elaborate grant applications that are common today, this request was concisely captured in twelve double-spaced pages that read in part:

The principal objectives of the pilot program as it is now envisioned can be set forth under five headings as follows:

1. To improve the effectiveness of the undergraduate instructional program of this College of Medicine and in so doing to provide a curriculum pattern which may prove beneficial to other colleges having similar characteristics . . .
2. To study the patterns of and needs for patient care as they pertain to health and professional personnel other than physicians and to determine how the faculty of the College of Medicine can best provide for the training and utilization of

these personnel within a program directed at the education of physicians . . .

3. To determine how our College of Medicine can best utilize, for objectives 1 and 2, the patient care institutions of this large medical center and how the College of Medicine can contribute to their present and future operations . . .

4. To determine how the College of Medicine can best utilize, for objectives 1 and 2, the other departments of the University of Illinois in Urbana and Chicago and how the College of Medicine in turn can contribute to their programs . . .

5. As a prerequisite to the foregoing objectives, to establish an organized and clearly identifiable center of educational research.

It is envisioned that this center, once it has been established, will be regarded as an essential unit of faculty organization and hence will be continued on a permanent basis.

When one examines the present-day complexities of medical education, medical and biological research and patient care programs, and when one gives full recognition to the potential strength to be gained by a medical school that is truly integrated into the university, one cannot escape the conviction that a permanent center or department of educational study and research is a necessity and not a luxury.

In this way the institutional stage was set for a major thrust in health professions educational research and development. It was apparently irresistible to the Commonwealth Fund Board of Directors, for at their next meeting in November they made an award of $112,000, the amount requested for a two-year study. It certainly proved irresistible to me when, in the course of the February 1959 AMA Congress on Medical Education, Granville Bennett described what he had in mind. Two visits and three months later I accepted the challenge, the excitement of which never lessened through seventeen years as program director.

Once committed, it was clear that my first task was to ensure a truly interdisciplinary endeavor, since experience had by then convinced me that neither those trained in medicine nor those trained in education could alone do what was required. The search for an associate program director, launched in the spring, was successfully concluded that summer when Lawrence Fisher agreed to accept the post. It proved to be a very sound choice. Fisher had been trained at the University of Chicago under Ralph Tyler (one of the top-rank-ing professionals in curriculum and evaluation), and he had already faced some of the problems of medical education as a consultant studying the internship in a general hospital. We both arrived on the Medical Center Campus in September to launch what was to become a pace-setting program, one that was alternately regarded with fondness and with resentment. It was called ORME—the Office of Research in Medical Education.

Both the charge given and the resources provided were different at Illinois from those at the Medical College of Virginia and at Stanford. The work here was to move toward the establishment of a permanent center, and the workers were to function as change agents, not merely as a new professional resource. This circumstance seemed to demand a different mode of operation, one that coupled responsiveness to faculty wants with initiatives designed to identify institutional needs and to stimulate action that would address them. It proved to be a difficult balance to achieve, because what faculty members generally seemed to want (clear and unambiguous answers about educational program organization or teaching methods) was often far from what the institution seemed to need (clarification of educational objectives and maximization of varied learning opportunities).

As long as the focus was on helping the faculty to do better what it was already doing (the responsive mode in work with individuals, departments, or committees), all went well; it was when probing initiatives suggested that unfamiliar alternatives might represent better educational strategies or instructional tactics that uneasiness appeared. The safeguard, recognized by all the players in this drama, was that ORME had no authority and only such power as the data and logic fed into decision-making groups could generate.

In order to avoid premature action, the work of the first year was organized chiefly around information gathering and dissemination. A substantial portion of time was spent in becoming familiar with the considerable number of faculty documents dealing with issues such as curriculum, instruction, examinations, admissions, and promotions, and in talking with faculty members, administrators, and students. The purpose of these efforts was to gain both understanding of the present state of things and insight into expectations and aspirations, always seeking from these sources some explicit delineation of objectives against which educational plans and activities could be cast. Equally important were the long hours we spent in classrooms, lecture halls, laboratories, clinics, wards, quiz sessions, and examinations, observing closely and documenting carefully the nature of the teaching-learning interaction, using the taxonomy of educational objectives created by Benjamin Bloom and his associates as a device for classifying the level of those exchanges.

As institutional learning goals began to emerge, small and focused studies were undertaken to illuminate the match between stated intent and actual performance: for example, the relationship between the faculty commitment to fostering critical thinking and their rating of academic achievement by students with demonstrably high and low levels of critical thinking skill (generally unrelated, but in some courses of instruction inversely related); the relationship between faculty concern for selecting students of high intellectual quality and the development of a school environment in which students with such quality could thrive (the match was limited).

Such findings, with as little judgmental overtone as could be managed, were reported back to individual teachers, departments, faculty committees, and larger groups both in the campus setting and during off-campus retreats. The purpose was to develop an agenda for action that could be taken *by the faculty,* given appropriate staff support by ORME. Probably the most significant result of these efforts was the gradual acknowledgment by a growing group of faculty leaders that less attention needed to be given to problems of staff teaching and more to those of student learning. As these explorations continued, it was becoming clear to many that it was not the specification of objectives, nor the organization of curriculum, nor the quality of instruction that had the most profound impact upon the nature of learning; rather it was the examination system. The system at Illinois, like that in most other medical schools at the time, seemed almost deliberately designed to defeat achievement of the program goals that were most widely espoused. Rewards generally went not to the students who were independent thinkers and critical analysts of complex problems, but to those best described as "dependent memory banks" who could produce on demand the solutions teachers had provided (being careful to match different solutions for the same problem to the individual bent of a faculty examiner).

As a result of these findings, the first major institutional change, fostered and supported by ORME but adopted and implemented through faculty action, was not a curriculum change in the conventional sense of altering the arrangement or content or sequence of courses; it was a curriculum change in the more significant sense of altering the climate for learning by modifying the system of student appraisal. For a contemporary reader who is well acquainted with the concepts of formative and summative evaluation, the idea of separating learning from certifying examinations may seem to be no great pedagogic advance. In 1960, however, it was a major step in the face of faculty skepticism that examinations that "didn't count" could serve any useful purpose (some still feel that way). Even today there will be many who recognize the difficulty of shifting responsibility for certification from individual departmental assessment of achievement in each discipline to institutional assessment of the way in which those separate parts are put together and used in solving problems that carry no disciplinary identification. Yet that too was achieved. Finally, through this process, came recognition that the task of creating examinations to probe the many cognitive, psychomotor, and affective goals of medical education is no work for amateurs, an outcome that legitimated the first expansion of ORME staff. The addition of experts in the field of tests and measurement provided both a service to the faculty and a stimulus to use examinations as tools for educational research as well as for academic judgment of student progress. The University of Illinois was fortunate that another of Ralph Tyler's former students, then in the examinations office at the University of Chicago, could be lured across the city first as a part-time consultant and later as a regular ORME staff member. Her name was Christine McGuire (Masserman).

Such a pattern of operation characterized the work of ORME during its developmental years. At the end of the pilot period (extended by an additional two-year grant from the Commonwealth Fund), the first *Report to the Faculty* included these summary observations:

> In working with Medical College faculty as individuals, departments or committees, the ORME staff has attempted to maintain a position of analytic detachment that would allow the observations reported and the suggestions made to be dealt with in an equally objective fashion. At the same time there has been no effort to conceal an educational philosophy often at odds with prevailing opinion in parts of the world of medical education. The coupling of a positive philosophy with an effort to be objective has, perhaps not unexpectedly, occasionally led

to questions about the sincerity of staff protestations that no hidden agenda was being pursued, that exploration (not manipulation) was the target. Faculty judgment on this issue must ultimately depend upon what is done rather than what is said. Thus the issue will not here be pursued beyond acknowledgement of the existence of this suspicion.

The persistent pattern of raising questions and offering help in *seeking* answers rather than *giving* them, although in keeping with the philosophical orientation of ORME, has also occasioned some distrust. It would have been far easier for faculty and staff alike had a one-year survey led to a specific proposal for a major or minor revision in course hours, content and sequence which could then have been discussed and accepted, modified or rejected by the faculty with a minimal expenditure of concern. It is this limited concept of curricular revision that the staff has attempted at all cost to avoid since experience at many levels of education has long demonstrated its ultimate futility. Neither a medical faculty nor its student body can afford to give precious time to fruitless manipulation of courses. Until basic questions of institutional climate are raised and pursued with diligence, the answers provided by mere shifting of hours serve little purpose beyond temporary solace. Thus ORME must continue to illuminate the questions, and be prepared to seek answers *with* faculty rather than *for* them. The progress that has been made in seeking such answers over this two-year period has to the ORME staff proceeded more rapidly than predicted. If to others it may seem snail-like, a review of the earlier pages of this document may provide some reassurance . . .

As the second biennium of its work begins, the Office of Research in Medical Education staff believes three questions should be considered and answered by the faculty to which it is responsible:

1. Is ORME moving in a manner in keeping with faculty understanding of purposes set out in the original document?
2. Should these purposes be modified or emphasis shifted during the continuing years?
3. Should the long-range opportunities be seized and developed?

Upon the thoughtful responses to these questions will the future be built.

Fortunately, the College Executive Committee endorsed the character of the program, the emphasis that had been established, and the importance of grasping the long-range opportunities. With this affirmation and support the pace quickened, and extramural as well as intramural challenges began to receive the attention of a slowly growing staff. But that stage will be depicted later.

PARALLEL DEVELOPMENTS

5

During the 1958-59 academic year, three medical schools established formal educational research and development programs. The two transplants from Buffalo have already been noted; a third blossomed independently in the fertile soil of north central Ohio.

No one even casually acquainted with the evolution of medical education needs to be reminded that Western Reserve University (now Case Western Reserve) was the site of a curriculum innovation that was more discussed, debated, and imitated than any other in the United States during the middle years of the twentieth century. The details of that dramatic tale will not be told here, but the events that led the Western Reserve faculty to establish a Division of Research in Medical Education as an integral element in the broader program are a significant part of this history.

When Joseph Wearn became dean in 1945, he inherited a school "facing problems of such serious import, that its survival as a first rate medical school was threatened"; an organization in which "each department was almost autonomous and planned its teaching with little or no consultation with other departments"; a faculty in which "many vacancies existed . . . due to age retirement, death, and resignations"; and a budget that was "wholly inadequate."[1] But in the spirit with which John Gardner later approached the unwieldy Department of Health, Education, and Welfare, Wearn regarded his heritage not as a set of insoluble problems, but as a collection of incomparable opportunities. And he went about the process of grasping them promptly.

Among the many things he did to transform the school, two stand out above all others. First, Wearn infected other people with his own spirit of high adventure. Through a skillful blend of enthusiasm and vision he was able to capture five new department heads in the first two years, five more in the next four years. These new leaders were "young, open-minded, and had no preconceived ideas of faculty structure. They entered readily and with enthusiasm into the major task of reappraisal of the curriculum and of teaching method."[2] Second, he managed to transform the faculty organization into one in which virtually all the teachers not only had an opportunity to participate in establishing educational policy and instructional procedures but also were expected to do so. Out of a loose confederation of baronies he created a democratic community whose members were committed to the achievement of a common goal: that of creating a first-rate school of medicine and a new educational program. After four years of study and debate this faculty felt ready to carry out the experiment in medical education that has won for Western Reserve a unique place in the academic pantheon.

To implement this work, Wearn imported from Harvard a respected internist, productive investigator, and gifted teacher, Thomas Hale Ham, who took up his post as coordinator of the contemplated new program in 1950. Significantly, this coordinator also continued his laboratory research and insisted on a regular tour of ward rounds at the Lakeside Hospital. It was equally significant that Ham avoided any direct affiliation with the dean's office, for like Wearn, he was committed to the view that education is the responsibility of a faculty, not of the administration. Thus when discussions reached the point of placing upon a faculty committee the specific responsibility for selecting and defining educational objectives, evaluating educational programs, and recommending instructional changes, Hale Ham was the natural choice to serve as chairman. It was a post from which he presided over the program for eight years.

Two principles served him as guidelines in this work, one drawn from a background in biomedical science, the other from an acquired educational philosophy. The first manifested itself in an unwavering spirit of inquiry about the soundness of what was proposed or instituted in the educational program, by an insistence upon the need to be as rigorous in looking at education as in looking at cells or molecules. The second was reflected in an unfailing reminder that *students* represented the central focus around which educational programs were built. This view was summarized in a 1962 report that said in part:

In planning "for the student" there is prime emphasis on the student, on his learning, and on learning in an increasingly effective manner. This principle has far-reaching effects because it places the educational needs of the student ahead of the convenience of the existing program of the faculty and ahead of the departmental structure or traditional sequence of subjects. It becomes possible and practical to consider the student's needs for a professional education and to explore ways to help him learn by himself by restructuring a program to fit his capacity, readiness, and pace.[3]

In the face of this orientation, it is probably not surprising that as early as 1956 the Committee on Medical Education proposed an independent Divison of Research in Medical Education (DORIME), nor was it unexpected that Ham should become the first director of DORIME when it was formally established in 1958. His first associates in this venture were two long-standing colleagues in the educational experiment: William R. Adams, a psychiatrist, and Milton J. Horowitz, a clinical psychologist who had already launched an in-depth study of selected medical students as they passed through this new educational program. In contrast to the Buffalo Project and its offspring, there were initially no staff members who would qualify as educationists. However, the need for this kind of expertise was soon recognized as the DORIME staff deliberated upon and planned future work. To fill this need they consulted with some of the most distinguished professional educators of the time: Ralph Tyler, Benjamin Bloom, Jerome Bruner, B. F. Skinner, Donald McKinnon, and T. R. McConnell, among others. Out of these discussions a major research and development focus emerged: education for problem solving in medicine. The General Faculty, to whom the proposal was submitted in 1960, endorsed this priority project, which became a central feature of DORIME's work for five years. Started as an intramural pilot study and designed in collaboration with a well-known educational research group at the University of Chicago, the project evolved into an elegant interinstitutional study that included both experimental and control schools. It also produced several admirable instructional volumes as well as a research report that surely added luster to the medical education literature.[4]

During an early phase of this work, the first full-time associates drawn from the world of education were added to the DORIME staff. Most of these educationists brought to the appointment a background and experience that reinforced the experimental stance that had characterized the initial team. But they were not an isolated or withdrawn group; as individuals and as a team they responded enthusiastically to requests for assistance in solving specific educational problems that troubled individual faculty members or groups of them. They supported fully DORIME's commitment to furthering educational innovation and enhancing the conditions that would optimize its achievement: "a receptive environment . . . a critical mass of people who were concerned . . . and an accompanying theory and evaluation."

Although each of the early efforts to apply educational principles in the setting of medicine included a research thrust, priority at Buffalo, the Medical College of Virginia, and Illinois was for action research, while that at Western Reserve more closely matched the experimental model. As Hale Ham later described it: "DORIME has been acting as a safety valve and guide to the faculty members as they perceive problems and try to work through the difficult process of creating solutions. Rather than allow that creative energy to remain pent up, DORIME provides the necessary support and guidance to channel it toward productive ends. It is a sanctuary to which the faculty can turn to reflect upon their educational problems."[5]

Sanctuary and reflection, comfortable support more than uncomfortable prodding: to an outside observer these were the qualities that seemed to characterize the early work of DORIME as it won internal acceptance and external respect.

At the University of Pennsylvania, Julius Comroe had worked his way up the academic hierarchy in the Medical School Department of Pharmacology, where good teaching was highly prized. It was his intense personal interest in improving basic science instruction that lay behind a small-scale, and regrettably short-lived, teacher training program at that institution. When Comroe became head of the Department of Physiology and Pharmacology in the university's Graduate School of Medicine, he set up an informal program designed to improve the quality of faculty lectures, and to provide for his graduate students, most of whom would become faculty members, some guidance in how to use this most prominent of instructional techniques.

He was stimulated to report this experience[6] after reviewing the results of a questionnaire circulated among those selected to participate in the 1953 AAMC Teaching Institute in Physiology, Biochemistry, and Pharmacology. When queried about whether teaching skills might be improved through instruction in the art of teaching, a majority of respondents replied affirmatively, although with varying degrees of enthusiasm. Even more astonishing was the fact that 72 percent expressed readiness to enroll in a course on teaching techniques that emphasized teaching basic medical sciences. However, this willingness was usually qualified by insistence that course leaders be faculty colleagues, not professional educators. It was just such a program that Comroe had already started.

The format he selected would today be called micro-teaching. Each faculty volunteer prepared a 15-minute lecture, which was delivered to peers. The peer group then engaged in a discussion of the lecturer's performance while the performer listened to an audiotape recording of what he had said (today the recording would be on videotape). The speaker then rejoined the group and shared with them a personal analysis of his own lecture; this was followed by reactions, comments, criticisms, and praise from the others. The group as a whole finally identified important aspects of the speaker's technique that needed improvement, and made a written record of these recommendations as a point of reference for the next round.

In sum, it was a self-help operation of the best kind. Even in the absence of professional leadership, these sessions succeeded in hastening the development of lecturing abilities in a number of those who participated. Unfortunately, as Comroe noted, the approach did nothing to improve other components of the instructional skills a teacher must employ. But it was a beginning, one that provided a base in experience for a part of the proposal he then made to the National Institute of Neurological Disease and Blindness for support of an ophthalmology-neurology academic training program. Two-thirds of the proposed training was to be in hard disciplines such as mathematics, statistics, physics, and chemistry, but the remaining third would be devoted to training in teaching, medical writing, and medical administration.

In the climate of 1954, probably no one except an academician with such unquestioned scientific credentials could have gained a hearing at the National Institutes of Health for such a scheme. Comroe not only got a hearing; he got a two-year grant to implement the program. Regrettably, it was put to the full test of practice only once, and with only twelve participants. Before it could be tried again, the organizer moved to the University of California Medical Center in San Francisco as founding director of the Cardiovascular Research Institute, and the program at Pennsylvania disappeared.

Although Comroe has continued to speak persuasively about the importance of training in teaching for medical school faculty members and has included an abbreviated experience of this kind in his postdoctoral training programs, it was not until 1977 that he fully acknowledged the possibility that professionals from the discipline of education might conceivably make a helpful contribution to such efforts.

At least one other North American medical school was also giving attention to faculty development, and in a manner not unlike that which had been undertaken at the University of Pennsylvania. A significant difference was that at the University of Saskatchewan a professional educator was involved from the beginning.

When Alexander Robertson was asked in 1958 to establish a Department of Social and Preventive Medicine at that medical school, he recognized the great challenge—which had rarely been met successfully—to capture student interest in this emerging discipline. His attack on the problem was twofold: developing a curriculum that required active student participation, and providing teachers with guidance in the skillful use of instructional methods that would foster such activity. The small group sessions selected to fulfill the first purpose were carefully designed to address explicit educational objectives; the second task was accomplished through independent observational analysis of what actually took place in those classrooms.

The observational team included a physician and a professional educator. Each class session was also tape-recorded to provide an objective point of reference for the critique they conducted the following day with all departmental teaching faculty members present. This was often a painful exchange, as teacher performance was cast against objectives, and pedagogic weaknesses as well as strengths were subjected to the penetrating light of analysis. Despite the discomfort engendered by these meetings, Robertson reported that "our group as a whole is convinced that it is only by such rigorous self-evaluation that a group of medical teachers can maintain their teaching skills in the same way as they would certainly wish to maintain their practicing and scientific skills: i.e., by a process of continuing education about education itself."[7]

It is sad to note that the Saskatchewan program, like the one at Pennsylvania, was never integrated into the institutional fabric. Following Robertson's departure to become director of the Milbank Fund, momentum was slowly lost, and soon nothing remained but a report and a memory.

The ferment in medical education during the late 1950s and early 1960s was by no means an exclusively North American phenomenon; that which was brewing in the United Kingdom, and in Latin America, is also a significant part of this evolutionary tale.

In its Second Interim Report, issued in 1955, the Medical Teaching Committee of the Royal College of Physicians called attention to the fact that "In the past ten years no country has produced so many wise reports on the improvement of medical education as Great Britain, and no country has done so little about it."[8] One of the key figures in changing this British posture was John Ellis, then an assistant physician at the London Hospital and sub-Dean of the London Hospital Medical College. That same year a Rockefeller Foundation grant made it possible for Ellis to study directly, or to discuss with representatives, the educational programs of twenty American medical schools, some stable, others in the midst of major curriculum change. His findings and reflections were reported in the Gouldston Lecture, first given before the Royal College of Physicians and later published in the *Lancet*. Among the conclusions he reached was a significant recommendation that one major step toward reform of medical education would be "to establish a means whereby it can itself be studied. Research is necessary in three things — in learning, in teaching, and in the pattern of medical practice."[9] Ellis went on to suggest that this need represented an unusual opportunity for collaboration between the Royal Colleges and the universities. Specifically, he called for the establishment of a National Council or an Institute on Medical Education.

And the time was nearly ripe to do so. In 1957, the General Medical Council, in a dramatic policy change, abandoned its century-old posture of prescribing minimal curriculum content to medical schools and licensing bodies, substituting general recommendations accompanied by encouragement for the schools to experiment with their curricula. This new permissiveness was just the stimulus needed to precipitate a coalescence of individuals and groups interested in the renovation of medical education into an organization that would facilitate communication among them, as well as promoting and conducting educational research. It was called the Association for the Study of Medical Education (ASME). John Ellis was its first secretary and executive officer.

The founders of this body felt it particularly important for the organization to be inclusive rather than exclusive, and from the beginning a varied membership was encouraged. It encompassed corporate bodies such as medical schools, Royal Colleges, medical institutes, regional hospital boards, and medical associations within the United Kingdom and throughout the British Commonwealth, as well as interested individuals — full-time or part-time teachers, administrators of health professions educational facilities, and medical practitioners. Although the Association was founded by physicians, and medically trained individuals were its major architects, an early effort was made to include persons whose background and training were in education itself. In fact, at the second annual conference of the Association (1959), which dealt with methods of learning and techniques of teaching, one of the major contributors was W. D. Wall, director of the National Foundation for Educational Research, who later became a member of the ASME executive council. This early collaboration with the educational establishment subsequently produced a joint course on educational objectives and methods and later encouraged the establishment, within the University of London Institute of Education, of a University Teaching Methods Research Unit that initially had a strong interest in medical education.

Many years passed before this kind of work became an integral part of the structure and function of a British medical school. In the interval, however, the Association, through its conference program, research projects, and later the *British Journal of Medical Education* (of which Ellis was the first editor), kept issues of medical teaching and learning, and of educational research and development, before the medical education community in much of the English-speaking world.

Like their counterparts in the United States and the United Kingdom, medical educators in Central and South America were also reexamining educational program objectives and practices. Encouraged and supported by the Pan American Health Organization (PAHO), the Kellogg and Rockefeller Foundations, and the Milbank Fund, three Latin American Conferences on Medical Education were held between 1957 and 1962. These meetings dealt primarily with the resources and facilities required for optimal education, the academic preparation and scientific qualifications needed by faculty members, the content and organization of medical school curricula, the choice of instructional methods, the need for additional instructional materials, the selection of medical students, and the problem of growing enrollments. The Declaration of Mexico, formulated during the first conference in 1957, addressed all these issues and served for many years as a kind of Magna Charta for Latin American medical educators.

At the second conference, held in 1960 at Montevideo, Uruguay, a significant reference to training medical teachers was included in the discussions. Among the recommendations that emerged from these deliberations was one urging the establishment of faculty training centers that would, in addition to ensuring the best scientific preparation of medical school staff, promote improvements in teaching. How this was to be done was not spelled out, but by then there already existed several Latin American programs that might have served as models.

For example, as early as 1956 the National University of Buenos Aires had both established the principle of requiring special training for physicians who planned to pursue a teaching career, and implemented a formal program to fulfill this objective. It was an ambitious offering that required five years to complete. First-year course work, which occupied several hours each week, dealt with the philosophy and history of science. During the second year, courses on pedagogic methods were given by professional educators. Upon completion of this classroom work, each candidate was required to present an original paper on a specific problem in medical education. The remaining three years were essentially work/study programs, with teaching assignments occupying roughly half the time and educational research activities filling the other half. Teaching assignments were reduced in the final year so that each candidate might become more familiar with other academic activities in the training department. Annual examinations were given, and a final evaluation determined whether the trainee would win recognition as an "authorized professor."

At the University of Chile in Santiago, Dr. Ramon Ganzarain and his associates had also been offering members of the medical faculty an opportunity for special training in medical education. Here the focus was on strengthening the human relationship between teachers and students as a means of improving the climate for learning. The work was later extended beyond this one institution in a form that became known as the Laboratory in Human Relations and Medical Teaching.[10]

The principal method of instruction in these laboratories (which ran six hours daily during the two-week session) was the Training Group, now generally known as a T-group. It was designed to demonstrate through a personal experience how issues such as role perception, struggle for leadership, authority models, and need for approval can impede learning, as well as how resolution of these conflicts can facilitate that process. This experiential method was supplemented by more content-oriented instruction through discussion groups built around readings on selected educational topics. Finally, participants engaged in a variety of skill exercises intended to increase their ability to comprehend and to manage the dynamics of group work.

Between 1962 and 1965 eleven such programs were offered in five Latin American countries by the original organizers and some of their students. It is interesting to note that Edward Bridge, who had planted the seed that grew into the University of Buffalo Project in Medical Education, was an early contributor to this parallel effort and was later engaged by the Pan American Health Organization to coordinate further extension of these Laboratory offerings. By the end of the decade nearly 1,200 medical school teachers had taken part in such programs.

Before this goal was achieved, however, the Latin American leaders repsonsible for the first two conferences on medical education had organized a third, held in 1962 at Viña del Mar, Chile. Here the proposal first made in 1961, to organize a Pan American Federation of Associations of Medical Schools, was adopted. Among the specific program components on which Federation sponsors agreed was one calling for "establishment of . . . advanced training centers for teaching personnel." Further amplification of the intent made it clear that emphasis would be given to training in the scientific aspects of medicine. An apprenticeship in teaching under established medical faculty members, not professional educators, was also to be included. As one observer pointed out, "There was no general agreement about the necessity for teachers to have formal training in pedagogy as a part of this preparation." However, when the Federation was formally activated at the Fourth Pan American Conference in 1964, the governing council and executive director accepted as one of their foremost tasks that of raising the professional level of medical educators, saying:

> Medical educators cannot be improvised and their efficiency does not depend merely on their clinical or scientific experience. Both are no doubt fundamental and should be evaluated objectively as to their quality and quantity. But they are not enough. Problems pertaining to the philosophy of education, the methods and techniques of the learning process, the programming of curricula and their supervision, the organization and administration of schools, and research in the specifically pedagogical aspects of University level teaching, requires special technical information and attention. Unfortunately, this background is not always found in individuals with a higher scientific and clinical skill in spite of their inclination toward teaching activities. In order to remedy the situation, the organization of several regional centers for advanced research training and instruction in teaching methods for medical educators is under way.[11]

But that development was part of a more general set of international repercussions, to be described in a later chapter.

Although the intent of this book is to explore the evolution of educational research, development, and teacher training in medicine, it would be chauvinistic to ignore parallel efforts in other health professions.

During the years with which this chapter deals, collegiate nursing programs were steadily displacing hospital-based training as the most respected path toward registration. As in other university divisions, the new nursing faculty members were expected to possess some academic qualification beyond a baccalaureate degree. But unlike most other university disciplines, there was then no well-established tradition of graduate education in nursing itself. A few nurses met the requirement for advanced training through graduate degree programs in the basic biomedical sciences; some won their academic credentials in public health; but the most popular path toward this goal was advanced education in education itself.

As a result, nursing faculties today probably have more individuals qualified in both the health field and in education than any of the other health professions. Yet an impartial observer of nursing education, or of the nursing education literature, is not likely to conclude that educational research and development have become a prominent feature of academic or professional nursing education. Certainly there have been no major institutional units or programs of educational research in nursing resembling those that have appeared in medicine.

In dentistry, things have been very different. Even though educational research, development, and teacher training may now be more thoroughly organized and institutionalized in medical schools, dental faculties had staked a claim and begun to mine the field of education long before physicians discovered the potential of this emerging science. As early as 1936, dental faculty interest in this work had reached such a pitch that the New York University School of Education, in collaboration with the College of Dentistry, established a Division of Dental Education and started a formal program leading to a graduate degree. That year also saw the Dental School and the Graduate School of Education at Harvard offer a two-week summer course on the principles of teaching and learning, with particular reference to dental student education. Although both programs seemed to represent the substantive response to a need clearly acknowledged by dental educators, they must have been premature: the program at NYU was discontinued in 1940, and the Harvard program was never repeated.

These innovations were an important beginning, however, and they provided useful models that encouraged others to initiate more modest efforts. Between 1937 and 1947, at least ten dental schools started some kind of faculty development program with the help of professional educators. For example, at Northwestern University a professor of education was recruited as a short-term consultant to the dental faculty; at the University of California, fifty dental school faculty members completed thirty hours of course work in educational psychology; at Howard, Columbia, Kansas City, and Temple, regular lectures on educational theory and practice were offered by experts drawn from their colleges of education; and at Indiana, Minnesota, and Oregon, in-service work/study programs were initiated.

A major contribution to this development was that made by the American Association of Dental Schools. The Curriculum Survey

Committee, appointed by the Association in 1930, launched a national study of how educational programs for dentistry were then organized and implemented. This was no casual investigation, but a serious endeavor conducted under the leadership of a full-time study director drawn from the world of higher education. Upon completing this task, and stimulated by what had been discovered, the committee turned its attention to the problems of teaching and learning in dentistry. Under the same leadership, a lengthy report was prepared that attempted to synthesize the potential application to dental education of then current educational theory and practice. Under the general title "Learning and Teaching Dentistry," seventeen segments were published serially in the *Journal of Dental Education* between 1941 and 1945. It was a remarkable achievement and served for many years as a significant reference for dental educators. Unfortunately, the work did not penetrate very deeply into the educational sensibility of other health professions.

By the late forties the time was ripe for another major institutional effort to exploit, in a concerted and continuing way, the experience that had now been gained. In 1948 the deans of dentistry and education at Temple University recognized this opportunity and jointly charged a committee drawn from both schools to determine how a collaborative program might be developed. The committee's first recommendation was for the initiation of a detailed study to identify the learning and teaching problems then existing in the Dental School. The study was to be comprehensive, was to include observational analysis of instruction as well as a survey of faculty and student views, and was to be carried out by a member of the education faculty.

This investigation produced a consolidated list of ten educational problems that required attention, and to which professional educators might make a significant contribution in terms of finding solutions. These issues became the basis for two faculty development programs that were planned and launched in 1950: one, a continuing weekly in-service seminar/workshop; the other, a formal graduate program leading to a master's or doctoral degree in dental education.[12] The movement in dentistry had now come full circle, and it anticipated by at least a decade what later occurred in medicine.

With further assistance from the Kellogg Foundation (already an important catalyst in these efforts), the extension of faculty development programs in dental schools continued through the development of regional conferences, the establishment of at least one other graduate program (at the University of Michigan), and the further elaboration of in-service training efforts. It is interesting to note that one of the most prominent among the latter programs was instituted in the College of Dentistry at the University of Illinois Medical Center, where at about the same time a major educational research and development unit was being established in the College of Medicine.

Despite the extent and variety of these activities, the Commission on the Survey of Dentistry in the United States found in 1961 that 85 percent of the dental faculty members responding to a questionnaire expressed a conviction that they would benefit from an in-service education program in dental teaching, but only 19 percent indicated that their schools offered such a training opportunity. This led the Commission to recommend that "Dental Schools develop or improve faculty in-service programs on the fundamental principles of teaching and the problems facing dental education."[13]

Apparently the need still had not been met.

GROWTH AND INFILTRATION

6

Between 1959 and 1962, interest in the work initiated at the University of Buffalo clearly quickened. This interest was generously nourished by members of the original Project in Medical Education staff and their new associates, who in various permutations and combinations seemed to float back and forth across the national landscape more like itinerant than resident educators in medicine.

Curiosity about what they had to say cropped up in many places. First of all were the medical schools. Some of the schools that had already introduced faculty conferences or retreats to discuss educational issues were now attracted by the fresh input that could be provided by this new breed of educational professional in medicine. Among such gatherings, extending from a few hours to a few days, in which the still small cadre took part were those held at the University of Pennsylvania, the Medical College of South Carolina, the University of Washington, the Albany Medical College, the University of Alberta, and the University of Rochester.

There were also special interest groups that used their professional association meetings to learn more about these unfamiliar "principles" of education. For example, the Association of Hospital Directors of Medical Education devoted two days to such a workshop; the American Academy of Microbiology, the American College of Radiology, and the Baltimore City Medical Society all set aside meeting time for such presentations; and the California Medical Association organized a special residential workshop at which those concerned with the continuing education of physicians could explore the implications of educational science to that portion of the educational continuum. Even agencies within the Federal establishment began to nibble. The National Institute of Neurological Disease and Blindness invited one of the new professionals in medical education to critique a day-long discussion of the training in otolaryngology being supported by the Institute; the Office of Vocational Rehabilitation asked a group of them to participate in planning and conducting a three-day national meeting on education in this field.

Perhaps most important at this stage was the catalytic contribution of the American Heart Association (AHA) made through its Committee on Professional Education under the prodding of Dr. Frederick Lewy (and later Dr. Richard Hurley), the staff member responsible for guiding and supporting the committee's work. The continuing education of practitioners was one of the committee's major concerns, and when in 1960 a special conference was called to develop an AHA position on this topic, several of those now identified with medical education research and development were included among the participants. The resulting report, *A Physician's Continuing Education,*[1] was in one respect a milestone: one-third of the content dealt with the process of learning, the principles of teaching and of program planning, and the importance of research in professional education. Among the eight recommendations made by the committee, five reflected an educational development/action research orientation. Attached to these conceptual proposals were specific dollar figures needed for support. Such a document, emerging from a respected voluntary health organization and from a committee whose members were predominantly distinguished academicians and practitioners, provided new momentum for a growing drive to introduce rational inquiry and scientific objectivity into the process of medical education.

Fortunately, the AHA initiative did not end with the publication of this report; funds were appropriated and actions followed. Two of those actions should be noted here (others will be discussed later). The first was a workshop on educational program planning and implementation, organized by the University of Illinois Office of Research in Medical Education for AHA committee members themselves and for professional staff in AHA affiliates who had direct responsibility for continuing education activities. The second action was a grant-in-aid program that made it possible for several medical schools to hold faculty retreats that were planned and conducted in collaboration with established medical education research units. Both the Hahnemann Medical College and the Ohio State University School of Medicine, the first two institutions to receive such grants, later created their own educational research and development programs.

However, the greatest boost to this new work came from the organization whose primary mission was the continuing improvement of medical education — the Association of American Medical Colleges.

By virtue of its constituency, if nothing else, the Association had been concerned with curriculum organization and instructional activities in medical schools since it was founded in 1876. Some of its early leaders were even advocates of the view that medical teachers needed to learn more about the principles of education if their efforts to prepare future physicians were to be maximally efficient and effective. Yet it is probably not unfair to say that in spite of such important projects as the successful introduction of a standardized procedure for assessing the academic qualifications of applicants to medical school, the dominant tone of the AAMC was that of an informal Dean's Club in which members gathered annually to exchange administrative experiences more than to explore with creative objectivity solutions to the academic problems that medical schools faced.

This quiet enclave, if such a description is accurate, was shattered in the turbulent years following World War II. The remarkable achievements of military medicine, and of the supporting biomedical research enterprise, had an impact on medical school programs that can only be likened to the one experienced in the post-Flexner years. The spirit of scientific inquiry that swept through basic science departments in the 1920s now engulfed clinical departments as well; and the public clamor for miracles and miracle workers was irresistible, particularly since the funds that made all this seem achievable began to flow in ever-increasing amounts from federal sources. It was inevitable that the Association would also change with the altered aspirations and needs of its institutional members. This new vigor made its appearance in the early 1950s and gained further strength with the appointment of a full-time executive director in 1957.

Ward Darley brought to this post an unusual combination of experiences. He had been a practicing internist, a professor of medicine, dean of a medical school, and finally president of the University of Colorado. Out of this background came a keen awareness of the need for change in medical schools and medical schooling if both were to fulfill their potential for elevating the quality of health services to a level that matched the rising expectations now evident on all sides. Darley had no master plan tucked up his sleeve and no intention of trying to impose on all schools a single pattern of operation. As a scholar whose vision had been sharpened by abrasive as well as informative encounters with many disciplines beyond medicine, he did recognize the pressing need to explore alternatives to the conventional wisdom about medical education as well as medical practice. He was particularly sensitive to the importance of determining the role that emerging social and behavioral sciences might play, in concert with well-established biomedical sciences, in the search for new solutions to old problems, not to mention the means for dealing with new ones.

The AAMC was ready to undertake such a new look; in fact, it had already started. In his 1952 presidential address, George Packer Berry described the critical reexamination of medical teaching to which the Association had committed itself. A major thrust in this exploration was to be a series of teaching institutes (Berry later referred to them as "national faculty meetings") that were envisioned as "instruments for helping us to extirpate from the curriculum what has become archaic, add what is new of significance, in order to restructure it around an essential scientific core consonant with advancing knowledge . . . [and] attempt to restructure the teaching program to accommodate comprehensive medicine without diminishing scientific medicine."[2]

With these general goals in mind, the first three teaching institutes, which dealt sequentially with the basic biomedical sciences, focused chiefly on curriculum content and organization. From the viewpoint of participants and sponsors alike the meetings were remarkably successful in providing both information and inspiration. From the viewpoint of professional educators, however, they may have seemed less so, since the discussion of educational processes (such as the derivation and specification of behavioral objectives, or the design of instructional strategies and evaluation tactics) was little more than an exchange of personal opinions and experiences rather than utilization of systematically developed data on these topics. But no professional educators were there to raise such questions, or if they were their voices were not recorded in the published reports.

Out of these three gatherings came a general realization that not enough was known about how to select students who could deal most successfully with the content of medical education, and a growing uneasiness that the climate for learning in medical schools might not be all that it should be. Thus the 1956 institute was devoted to the issue of selection, and that in 1957 to the institutional environment. For the first time social and behavioral scientists (in the form of clinical and experimental psychologists) were introduced into both the planning committees and the institute deliberations. The result was electrifying. As George Berry later described it:

> At the Institute the psychologists marshaled experimental evidence providing exciting glimpses into the vast but as yet still largely unexplored domain of "interest" and "motivation." They showed how one could study objectively the non-intellectual characteristics of man that so dominate the uses that are made of intellectual endowment. Thus the 1956 Institute reached a milestone in the recognition that psychology has produced insights into the mosaic of personality that have profound implications for the future of medicine.
>
> Beyond this achievement at the 1956 Institute is the promise that continuing mutual efforts of psychologists, medical teachers, and scientists will eliminate any barriers between psychology and medicine and replace them with a dynamic interface. This replacement was indeed achieved at Colorado Springs. It puts in prospect a major advance in medical education in our time.[3]

The following year, sociologists and a few professional educators had their turn as planners and participants and were equally well received.

As an officer of the Association, Darley had taken part in several of these Teaching Institutes and shared with other members of the AAMC Executive Council a sense of pride in what they had achieved. Nonetheless, he recognized that other tactics and strategies for further improving the quality of medical education could not be neglected. Originally he was somewhat skeptical about the potential contribution of professional educators to the achievement of such a goal. However, correspondence with the Buffalo group, which was initiated in 1957 shortly after his assumption of the executive directorship, further conversations with Stockton Kimball, who was then treasurer of the Association, and a visit to the Project in Medical Education early in 1958 led to a change of heart and ultimately to

Darley's enthusiastic support of this work. The first major manifestation of this posture was his endorsement of the proposal that the first Summer Institute on Medical Teaching, in June 1958, be jointly sponsored by the University of Buffalo and the AAMC.

When in 1959 I moved from the University of Buffalo to the University of Illinois, the geographic proximity of the College of Medicine's Office of Research in Medical Education in Chicago to the AAMC executive director's office in suburban Evanston shortened the lines of communication between us and strengthened the professional relationship that Darley and I had by then established. Our informal discussions about further collaboration beyond joint conduct of summer seminars led, in December 1959, to a long memorandum outlining a five-year plan of action, which I prepared at Darley's request. The proposal called for continuation of the summer seminars on medical education directed to a national audience, in 1960 and 1961; the establishment of regional seminars in 1961, 1962, and 1963 at which the focus would be on the special educational concerns of a small group of geographically related medical schools (each seminar to be preceded and followed by staff visits to the involved institutions); and the development of individual school seminars on medical education in 1962, 1963, and 1964. The draft was later expanded to include the initiation of fellowships in medical education, lasting from three to twelve months, for both medical faculty members and professional educators; special workshops on selected educational topics in connection with AAMC annual meetings; a similar series of workshops for individual schools; and intensive institutional self-study programs leading to intramural seminars on medical education.

These suggestions were forwarded to the AAMC Executive Council in January 1960 with a covering memorandum from Darley noting that "it was the need for AAMC activity in the area of the Buffalo type of development that I had in mind when I prepared part of my . . .paper 'The Next Ten Years and the Association of American Medical Colleges.' " Following extended discussion, the Executive Council approved sponsorship of a 1960 summer seminar with the University of Illinois and requested the Committee on Research and Education to review the proposals and recommend what the Association should be doing to supply leadership in these areas.

The 1960 seminar was different in only one significant respect from those that had preceded it: for the first time the staff included a person who had not been part of the original Buffalo team. He was, however, someone who would play a central role in the further extension of educational research and development in medicine. Paul Sanazaro was at the time an associate professor of medicine at the University of California Medical Center in San Francisco. He had been a participant in the 1959 Summer Institute, had served with Stephen Abrahamson on the staff of a West Coast educational workshop, and had just published a provocative paper entitled "The Placebo Effect in Medical Education," in which he said among other things:

> The influence of the student-teacher interaction has been generally underestimated in evaluating new curricular designs, much as the placebo effect may obscure truth in clinical therapy. In medical education proper application of "placebo factors" may be beneficial; but misdirected placebo therapy is always dangerous for it obscures the basic defect and delays application of specific therapy.
>
> Without in any sense detracting from the value and importance of curriculum analysis and experimentation I would suggest that a greater immediate benefit would result from instruction of faculty members in the principles and techniques of effective teaching. Provision for this should be a faculty elective. This may not affect senior faculty members since willingness to be taught and faculty seniority are reported to be inversely proportional. The Project in Medical Education begun at the University of Buffalo may help define constructive approaches to this problem. Ideally the Association of American Medical Colleges should eventually function as a central resource center for schools wishing to initiate such programs.[4]

The executive director was prepared to move in the direction suggested by Sanazaro, but there was still skepticism among some AAMC leaders that any major effort of this kind would pay significant dividends. In order to gain some independent assessment of such a program's potential worth, two of these leaders were asked to serve as participant observers at the 1960 summer session. Dr. George Aagaard, dean of the University of Washington School of Medicine and president-elect of the AAMC, summarized their positive response to the experience in an editorial entitled "Pedagogy in Medical Education," which appeared in the April 1961 *Journal of Medical Education*. This public acknowledgment of merit, and of the need to extend such work, was a significant element in preparing the ground for another step in AAMC program development.

It was not as though the Association had completely neglected educational research and development. Since the early 1950s, under one label or another, there had been some organizational entity comparable to the Division of Research, which was at the time thriving under the direction of Helen Hofer Gee. This division had provided staff support and assembled the impressive data upon which the deliberations of Teaching Institute participants were based. The division staff had also embarked upon a major study of the intellectual and nonintellectual characteristics, medical school performance, graduate training experience, career choice, and professional activities of the class of 1960 in more than a score of carefully selected schools. The Division of Operational Studies, under the direction of Lee Powers, was equally productive, documenting the nature and variety of fiscal and administrative characteristics of American medical schools and their teaching hospitals. The time was now ripe for establishing a comprehensive Division of Educational Studies to address issues of curriculum, instruction, and evaluation in medical education programs and the relationship of educational experiences to the quality of health care provided by medical graduates and postgraduate trainees.

The general outline of purpose and activities for such a unit within the AAMC headquarters structure was developed in a series of internal memorandums and was further elaborated in communications between Ward Darley and various foundation executives, since external support would surely be required to extend the work already undertaken and to mount the additional initiatives now contemplated. For example, the correspondence with Thomas Parran, then president of the Avalon Foundation, developed this proposal in the context of problems that medical schools then faced and the kinds of assistance that both the schools and the AAMC would need if they were to address these issues. The exchange with John Gardner, president of the Carnegie Corporation, culminated in a December 1961 proposal entitled "The Association of American Medical Colleges and the Need and Timeliness for Encouraging Research in Teaching and Learning in Medical Schools." As a summary statement of where this work fitted into the historical context and future perspective of medical education, Darley's proposal was remarkably perceptive and illuminating. It read in part:

For fifty years, American medical education has followed the path pointed out in 1910 by Abraham Flexner, who had a vision of the excellence that could be achieved by a profession based in the life of a university and built upon a solid foundation of scientific research. The accomplishments of these years are self-evident but the conflicts that have grown with them are only now emerging with a clarity that demands attention. For a mounting uneasiness is abroad that as medical schools have expanded and grown rich in full-time faculty of immense skill there has been a fractionation of the program of instruction and an increasing preoccupation with the subject matter of more and more highly specialized and increasingly isolated disciplines. Thoughtful critics on many sides are raising penetrating questions about the duration of medical education, its content and its ultimate effect upon the student as well as upon medical care for individual patients.

Such questions have provoked many imaginative curricular revisions during the last ten years. These changes have attempted to focus student and faculty attention upon the ultimate unity of the disciplines gathered together in the name of medical education and upon the patient to whom medical education is finally addressed. The rearrangements have sometimes shortened, sometimes lengthened the years of study but all have been created with the intent of making more profitable the student's investment of time and effort.

Bold and imaginative as these changes have been, they have seldom kept pace with the spirit of research that has in most other respects permeated the contemporary medical school. They have rarely been built upon, or even acknowledged the existence of, an immense body of information accumulated during the last half century through research in education. They have for the most part been derived from traditional principles of teaching rather than contemporary knowledge of learning. Described as educational experiments, they have rarely been developed with an experimental design: they have more often been offered as answers to implicit questions than as hypotheses worthy of testing.

The time has come to illuminate the educational issues medical schools must face realistically; to capitalize upon the professional wisdom and skills of those who have studied most carefully the principles upon which education must be built; and to establish the worth of research in medical education if sound conclusions, rather than strongly held opinion, are to guide us into the future.

Medical education does not face these problems alone. All university divisions and all institutions of higher learning would profit from the kind of searching examination envisioned here. There are few who have conducted curricular studies using the methods of science. Even the schools of education appear to have built their programs upon tradition rather than evidence, although their course of instruction is designed to teach students to do otherwise. Fortunately the scientific tradition built into medicine during the last fifty years, coupled with a current concern for its educational offerings, has provided the happy combination of circumstances and individuals that could lead the entire university community in a critical re-examination of education through sound and critical exchange of data.

If knowledge now emerging from medical research is to be fully utilized in medical practice, then it will be necessary to establish more effective ways of teaching that will lead to more efficient ways of learning. If the scientific method is to contribute to improved instruction, then educational goals must be scrutinized with scientific objectivity, instructional tools selected with scientific precision, and evaluation instruments developed with scientific accuracy. If these efforts are to be kept within the limits of academic capacity, they must be based upon a sound understanding of the intellectual and non-intellectual characteristics of faculty and students alike.

In such a new look at medical education, the Association of American Medical Colleges hopes to play a leading role as it works closely with schools now engaged in such efforts and encourages others to accept the challenge.

Darley then went on to describe the AAMC activities that made a move in this direction particularly timely and to outline in general terms the work contemplated for the proposed Division of Education. It must have been a persuasive document, for the result was an award from the Carnegie Corporation of $300,000 to get on with the task.

By the time the grant was officially accepted a project director had already been identified. At the November 1961 Teaching Institute, Darley first suggested to Paul Sanazaro that this directorship might be a post that would match Sanazaro's growing interest in the process of medical education and its impact on health care. The match proved to be compatible and the arrangements mutually agagreeable. In April 1962 the appointment was announced, and in July the program was launched. The general principles and specific

proposals that guided the development of the new division were presented to AAMC members at the next annual meeting of the Association in October 1962. Even before he could get his thoughts in
order, however, Sanazaro became the central figure in two collaborative activities whose origins preceded his appointment.

The first project was an extension of the Summer Seminars on
Medical Teaching. An earlier suggestion that this program might
be changed from a national group offering to a single-school activity
was picked up by Dean Arden Miller, who proposed that the University of Kansas Medical School be the site of such a pilot effort. Conceptually, the difference between the old and new thrusts was not so
much one of content as of focus. Questions of learning dynamics,
student attitudes and values, curriculum organization, instructional
methods, and evaluation procedures would still be dealt with, but in
the context of specific concern, problems, and opportunities within
an individual school. Such an orientation obviously demanded a different planning process. Members of the school faculty and administration, as well as AAMC staff and selected consultants, would
need to be involved in identifying the most promising topics for consideration and in accumulating school data that would serve as a
point of departure, or a point of reference, for seminar deliberations.

The planning group that was finally selected included representatives of the University of Kansas, who provided a channel of continuing communication with the medical school faculty and student
body; staff members from the AAMC, who accepted primary responsibility for the accumulation of required background data; and
consultants from the University of Illinois, who later served as the
principal seminar leaders. During four months of intermittent discussion this group reached agreement on site, format, and substance of the meeting; arranged special studies of personal values
and of critical thinking skills among University of Kansas medical
students (to illustrate with concrete local data an approach to eluci-
dation of these two troublesome academic questions); and requested
from the AAMC data bank national norms and a University of Kansas profile on institutional variables such as student aptitudes, attitudes, and career plans, the climate for learning, the source and
amount of income, and the allocation of expenditures.

The week-long residential conference held in June 1962 produced
a mixed response from forty medical faculty participants who

moved en masse from Kansas City to the parent university campus at Lawrence. Terminal assessments ranged from "Your program was one of the most provocative I have ever attended" to "I do not believe it a good idea, particularly for your staff, to conduct seminars for members of a single faculty." Overall the reaction was favorable, and was perhaps best summarized by an originally skeptical major department head who later wrote, "I did gain a great deal from your session and I am positive from conversation with other people that this was the general reaction of our entire group . . . Let me tell you from the bottom of my heart that I really appreciated your conference and any skepticism I might have had about it last winter is completely gone." Despite such a favorable summary there is little question that the experience left at least a few bruises on both sides, for the same writer also noted in his commendatory letter, "I have never attended a conference . . . in which there seemed to be such a general attitude of hostility . . ."

It was difficult then, and it remains so now, to be sure of what went wrong in the process, even though the product seemed to be satisfactory. One observer suggested that this faculty may have been unduly sensitized to implied criticism of their medical educational program by *Boys in White,*[5] a not always flattering sociologic study of the student/faculty culture in that medical school, which had appeared so recently. Another concluded that the visiting staff not only had been insufficiently sensitive to internal conflicts, which occasionally surfaced during the meeting, but also had underestimated both the knowledge that at least a few participants brought with them and the local work already done in applying some of the principles under discussion. Whatever the reason for what sometimes seemed more like an adversary than a collegial relationship, sponsors and staff alike learned that a seminar for the faculty of a single school is very different from one dealing with comparable content but offered to representatives of many schools. Out of this discovery came a substantially modified format for the programs offered in four subsequent years.

Paul Sanazaro described these intramural seminars on medical education as an effort to merge the purposes and principles of the Summer Institute programs developed at the University of Buffalo with those of the institutional self-study programs developed by regional accrediting commissions on higher education. The procedure finally adopted began in an interested school with the appointment

of a planning committee, of manageable size yet representing faculty and administration, senior and junior teachers, basic and clinical
scientists, full-time and voluntary staff, policy makers and those
who implemented policy. The local planning group took responsibility for selecting those elements of the educational program that
would be subjected to special study, securing cooperation from students and faculty in carrying out the necessary investigations, choos-
ing the seminar site and participants, and sharing leadership of the
seminar itself. Once the special study topics had been identified,
consultants in medical education research were recruited by the
AAMC to assist the committee in determining the most feasible
techniques for obtaining desired information about the school itself,
as well as comparative data on anonymous peer institutions. After
the local committee was appointed, a minimum of one year was
needed to complete the planning, to gather the data, and to prepare
for the culminating event, a week-long residential seminar for thirty
to forty invited participants. Throughout this period the planning
committee kept the faculty at large informed of what was happening and of what was to come in order to heighten their interest and
secure their support.

This activity was invariably an exhausting but exhilarating experience for the core group of AAMC Divison of Education staff members (Paul Sanazaro, Edwin Hutchins, William Sedlacek, Mary Lit-
tlemyer), the regular panel of consultants (Stephen Abrahamson,
Lawrence Fisher, Hilliard Jason, Christine McGuire, George Miller), other temporary consultants, and the planners/participants
from the four schools in which seminars were held: the University of
Maryland, Ohio State University, Tulane University, and the Medical College of Georgia. The methods of study, the process of program organization and implementation, the content, and the outcome of this work were described in Sanazaro's report entitled *Educational Self-Study by Schools of Medicine*. Ward Darley proudly
referred to this program as "one of the most significant recent developments within the AAMC."

But Sanazaro also inherited the embryonic plan for what may
have been an even more significant contribution to this educational
research and development effort, one that has certainly had a far
longer half-life than the intramural seminars.

The seed was planted by Hale Ham, director of the Division of
Research in Medical Education at Western Reserve. In January

1962, he proposed to Dr. Donald Anderson, then president of the AAMC, that "report meetings" be scheduled during the annual general meeting so that those doing research in medical education could share their findings with interested colleagues (Ward Darley, with his customary prescience, had anticipated this development in his 1961 request to the Carnegie Corporation for funds to support a Division of Education). After some hesitation the Executive Council endorsed the Ham proposal and designated as preliminary planners Donald Anderson (AAMC president), Robert Glaser (chairman of the Committee on Education and Research), Hale Ham, and George Miller; and from the AAMC staff, Ward Darley and Paul Sanazaro. This group was to "plan, organize, and conduct the first meeting. On the basis of experience (gained in the initial round) the Council expects that the committee will recommend a plan for its annual continuation as an integral part of the Association's development program of research in medical education." In March 1962 the ad hoc group recommended members of a regular planning committee, to include Hale Ham (chairman), John Ginther, Milton Horowitz, George Miller, George Reader, Edwin Rosinski, and Paul Sanazaro; later Winslow Hatch of the U.S. Office of Education was added. In April the Executive Council approved the recommendation; in May the meeting was announced and a call for papers was made; by July forty-one abstracts had been received; and on October 31, during the annual meeting held that year in Los Angeles, sixteen papers were presented and discussed in two sessions separated by a midday address entitled "Evaluation and Prediction" given by Benjamin Bloom.

Thus the annual Conference on Research in Medical Education (RIME) was born. The temporary committee that planned the initial program was shortly made a standing subcommittee of a parent group, significantly renamed the Committee on Research *in* Education (replacing the earlier designation Research *and* Education). From its beginning the annual RIME meeting has been a thriving enterprise, steadily attracting more interest and constantly aiming for higher research standards. In fact, the persistent push for better quality led at one point to a protest that "naturalistic" studies were being eliminated from consideration because of the planning committee's concern for academic and statistical rigor. Wisely recognizing the varied backgrounds, experiences, and orientations brought to this research meeting by an ever-expanding group of participants, the planners long ago gave up the single-program format. In fact, this diversity of interests and contributions made it necessary in 1977 to schedule multiple simultaneous meetings (twenty in all) to allow presentation and discussion of forty-eight papers, four poster sessions, and eight symposia on topics of special interest.

During the early years, papers presented at the conference were included in a special Proceedings published in the *Journal of Medical Education*. Later only the abstracts appeared there. Now the number of papers has grown so large that a separate publication appears each year just before the conference is held. This document has achieved such stature that since 1978 all accepted contributions have been included in the *Index Medicus*. Thus has the literature of medical education research, which was virtually nonexistent twenty years ago, come to maturity.

These manifestations of national interest in medical education research and development were important factors in gaining greater visibility for the work, and greater legitimacy as well. However, replication of the original institutional units at Western Reserve, the Medical College of Virginia, and the University of Illinois (all established in 1958-59) did not occur until 1962. When it did take place the site was another small upper New York State school, the Albany Medical College. Whether the relationship was causal or adventitious, this had also been the site of an earlier faculty retreat in which some of the original Buffalo Project in Medical Education team had taken part. A more immediate link with those origins, however, was the program director, Frank Husted, who came to Albany from Buffalo where he had been one of Abrahamson's graduate students.

One of Husted's significant contributions, made during a relatively short tenure, was the establishment of a seminar series on educational process for hospital residents. These house officers carry a major responsibility for teaching medical students but are rarely given any systematic preparation for the role.[6] Booked as a pilot venture, the seminars achieved modest success in enhancing the participants' teaching skills, but more importantly, perhaps, they provided significant new insight into the way such an introductory exercise for residents might be carried out more effectively in a subsequent round. But before he had a chance to repeat this program (or at least to report it), Husted moved on to try his talents and experience in a new federal initiative — the Regional Medicine Programs.

The Albany unit continued for several years under new leadership (another of Abrahamson's graduate students) but ultimately disappeared as an identifiable programmatic activity.

The next organized institutional unit appeared in 1963. The Division of Research in Medical Education (DRME) at the University of Southern California soon established itself as one of the leading American centers for this work, a position it continues to occupy. An important reason for the Division's longevity and success is the continuous leadership provided by Stephen Abrahamson, who was lured back to the West Coast by then dean Clayton Loosli. Although accorded divisional status, the unit was not initially blessed with a very substantial budget. Nevertheless, by operating in much the same fashion that he had used earlier at Stanford, Abrahamson managed to establish himself quickly as a competent and responsive resource to the faculty. In fact, this responsive stance has characterized the work of the Division ever since that modest beginning. In his first annual report Abrahamson noted that "the work which we have done more or less at the invitation of departments seems to me the area in which we should continue to put a major portion of our efforts." Reaffirming this posture one year later, he added, "While activities of this kind seldom result in major institutional changes, they nevertheless tend to influence quite significantly the total effort of the institution."

It was a technique of infiltration rather than confrontation. A review of the list of activities undertaken by the newborn division during the first eighteen months could leave little doubt that they would have widespread repercussions, if for no other reason than that so many faculty members were being stimulated to discuss questions of examinations and grading, curriculum organization and instructional alternatives, course evaluation and teaching skills from a new perspective. The work with individuals and departments was further reinforced by input to faculty committees such as those responsible for admissions and curriculum. Although the intensity of this work within the School of Medicine delayed the fulfillment of a desire for integral involvement with the School of Education, a linkage at least was established from the start. Abrahamson was given academic appointments in both schools; he was invited to conduct a graduate seminar on education for the professions; and he offered research assistant opportunities in DRME to graduate students in education.

But a responsive stance did not imply an absence of initiative.

The 1964 DRME Director's report went on to say, "In the year ahead I hope to be able to continue the pace in consultant services to departments and to members of the faculty. In addition I hope we are enabled to encourage the faculty to consider other broad areas for review . . . The one area in which I hope to see a truly major expansion of our efforts is that of teaching educationists to assume contributing roles in medical education."

These were ambitious aspirations for a new division in which the staff consisted of a director and one half-time graduate student, which functioned without a formal budget, and which after only one year of operation now faced an unanticipated change in medical school administration. Fortunately the new dean (Dr. Roger Egeberg) proved to be in every way as supportive of this young program as his predecessor had been.

To achieve the broader goals now envisioned demanded more funds than even the most supportive dean could mobilize from internal sources. Although initial efforts to attract external support were discouraging, by 1965 two major grants had been won, and their implementation propelled the USC Division of Research in Medical Education to a prominence that could scarcely have been predicted two years earlier. The project that excited greatest attention — SIM I, the computerized trainer for anesthesiologists (see Chapter 7) — grew out of earlier work with the Department of Anesthesiology on a plan for residency training. The second grant, to support production of a single-concept film series on the neurologic examination and the development of programmed patients as instructional aids, also served as a launching pad for the creative new career of a neurologist named Howard Barrows.

Not until 1965 was another medical education unit established. It became the first program (other than Western Reserve) in which the director had not been a participant in, or directly influenced by, the original University of Buffalo Project in Medical Education. Located at the Medical College of Georgia, it was headed by Loren Williams, who later moved to the Medical College of Virginia to build upon the heritage left by Edwin Rosinski.

There remained one major figure still to emerge from the seminal work at Buffalo. Hilliard Jason graduated from the University of Buffalo School of Medicine in 1958. Following an internship at the Buffalo General Hospital, he went on to a residency in psychiatry at the University of Rochester. During this period of specialty training he completed the dissertation that won him a doctorate in education as well. There followed two years at McGill University in Montreal where, in addition to clinical work, Jason also carried out an observational analysis of teaching practices in the Departments of Medicine and Surgery[7] (modeled after the one done as part of the Buffalo Project), which was the first such study conducted in a Canadian medical school. He returned to Rochester in 1963 as assistant professor of psychiatry and of education, and associate in medical education, to establish there the sixth program of educational research and development in a North American medical school. Although many activities were initiated in Rochester during his relatively short tenure, the one most widely known was the establishment of a national Clearinghouse of Programmed Instructional Materials in Medicine, a project facilitated by the series of national conferences on this topic that Jason organized and chaired. But it was the invitation to establish yet another educational research program that provided the opportunity for him to make a distinctive mark in the field.

When Andrew Hunt was selected as the founding dean for the Michigan State University College of Human Medicine, he brought to that task a firm commitment to make this new school different. Having worked closely with Stephen Abrahamson during the year he spent at Stanford, Hunt was convinced that he needed the help of someone professionally skilled in educational program planning, implementation, and evaluation. General support for this view and expression of willingness to cooperate were given by his counterpart in the MSU College of Education, but Hunt also wanted a resource that was an integral part of the medical school.

Once more Lester Evans served as an advisor and counselor in breaking new educational ground; and once again the Commonwealth Fund provided financial assistance for establishing what was to become the Office of Medical Education Research and Development (OMERAD). After consulting with several individuals already prominent in the field, Hunt invited Hilliard Jason to become the first director of the new unit and, perhaps not incidentally, the first physician appointed to the faculty.

It was Hunt's intention and Jason's desire that OMERAD should be a vital part of the faculty, both functionally and organizationally. To ensure this status it was established as an independent unit rather than as an arm of the Office of the Dean. Although the initial budget provided only two academic positions, plus support for two part-time graduate students, a major effort was made to involve a faculty member from each academic department in the work of OMERAD to such an extent that a joint appointment would seem mutually desirable. Insinuation of this unfamiliar resource into all program planning, implementation, and evaluation was thus assured. OMERAD was also represented in all major educational policy committees so that the views of professional educators would always be heard in the deliberations that preceded decisions. The number of these professionals whose views were available was further increased as the policy of joint appointments crossed college boundaries. Soon such well-respected individuals as Lee Shulman and Norman Kagen in the College of Education had also been enticed to become part-time members of the OMERAD staff.

This was clearly a unique collaborative endeavor, the first time that biomedical content and educational process experts had jointly planned a medical school curriculum from the beginning. Hunt's commitment to the principle and Jason's mobilization of the resources represented an enviable partnership. Out of the resulting interaction among individuals and groups came a program that emphasized individualized learning and student responsibility for achieving defined professional competence, de-emphasized conventional grades and grading, highlighted the attitudinal goals of medical education and the interpersonal skills that are essential in the delivery of optimal health care, and fostered achievement of these goals by incorporating early clinical experience and giving equal emphasis to social/behavioral and biomedical sciences.

In addition to participating in the creation of an innovative educational program for medical students, OMERAD was also charged by the dean with the "primary obligation of designing and implementing a longitudinal study that will provide measures of student progress with respect to program objectives . . . This unit will [also] be involved in a number of more delimited studies and carry out significant research in medical education that will have relevance beyond our program." The Office was further expected to develop degree and nondegree programs for those anticipating careers in medical education. In short, OMERAD was to fulfill all the obligations of an academic department, although whether it should be given official departmental standing has been a matter of periodic discussion and debate. Initially it was agreed that the less formal arrangement provided most of the advantages and few of the disadvantages of departmental status, but the discussion has not yet ended.

Reflecting on the role of OMERAD in the growth and development of the College of Human Medicine, the founding dean made these significant observations in 1977: (1) the presence of such an office and of its well-known director was a positive factor in faculty recruitment, particularly of the new group of clinicians that had to be attracted if the program goals were to be achieved; (2) the generally acknowledged reputation that has been won by the college is in no small measure a reflection of the contributions made by OMERAD to the educational philosophy and instructional practices within the school, as well as to the wider field of educational research and development; and (3) given another opportunity, he would certainly include such an educational resource as an early and integral component in the development of a new school.

Thus by 1966 the programs generally recognized as the big three among medical school educational research and development units (Illinois, Southern California, and Michigan State) had been firmly established. Their presence and their contributions certainly encouraged the establishment of other programs at a pace that accelerated during 1967 and 1968 and, after a brief plateau, spurted once more in the early 1970s. The pattern is shown in Table 6.1, but the forces that nourished this growth and development cannot be illustrated so simply. That story will require another chapter.

TABLE 6.1. New Medical Education Research and Development Units in the United States and Canada

Years	No. of Units
1957-1961	3
1962-1966	5
1967-1972	30
1973-1977	22

MOBILIZING SUPPORT

7

Without the generous support given to the earliest medical education research and development units by the Commonwealth Fund, it
is unlikely that the emerging science of education would have gained
the foothold that was achieved in a few medical schools by the mid-
1960s. But no realist among the early band of innovators could expect such support to continue indefinitely. All soon realized that if
the research and training activities implicit in their work were to
flourish, both institutional funds and additional extramural grants
would be required.

Fortunately, the growing interest in this field appeared at a time
of general expansion in the medical education establishment, a fact
that may have minimized any feeling of serious competition for
funds by well-established biomedical disciplines. However, it did
not lessen the intensity of conflict over whether this new thrust,
which clearly represented a challenge to the conventional wisdom
about medical schooling, was worth supporting at all. The initial
battle for sustenance was ultimately won, but the war over worth
still breaks out at unpredictable moments and in unexpected places.
If this account of experiences in the battlefield seems unusually personal, it merely reflects the inescapable truth that the number of
battlers was still small.

In keeping with academic practices at the time it seemed very natural to turn first to federal sources for assistance, particularly to that
most prominent source, the National Institutes of Health, where
Julius Comroe had found support for his faculty development program. But a director of research in medical education could not
command the same attention there as that accorded such a distinguished biomedical scientist as Comroe. This is not to suggest that

NIH staff members were unavailable or unwilling to listen. Although some of them may have questioned whether there was a legitimate science of education that could be applied to medical training programs, few denied the importance of giving more attention to the process of educating physicians and to the elements of medical teaching. However, importance of a topic does not necessarily make it a part of the NIH mission. Support of biomedical research and research training in the categorical areas defined by individual institute names was their concern. Responsibility for educational re search, the message went, belonged to other agencies of the federal establishment and particularly to the U.S. Office of Education.

Unfortunately, staff members in that Office saw the situation somewhat differently. Although they did have a legitimate interest in the study of vocational and technical education, and in the more general aspects of higher education, an ill-defined but nonetheless impenetrable curtain seemed to be drawn across those parts of the spectrum that dealt with science and health. In the matter of training educational research workers, USOE support mechanisms seemed to be limited to preparing those with general academic interests rather than the more specific and pragmatic concerns of an applied discipline such as medicine. These areas, many spokesmen suggested, were more properly in the domain of the National Science Foundation or the National Institutes of Health. Although it was difficult to be sure, the impression was strong that this conclusion did not represent a statutory requirement but a policy distinction that gave higher priority in the Office of Education to the more widespread and demanding problems of elelmentary and secondary schools.

National Science Foundation staff members were also approachable and generally sympathetic. In the end, however, their conclusion resembled that of the other agencies: medical education research, development, and teacher training belonged to someone else. Specific educational research project proposals that fell within NSF priorities would not be rejected because they came from medical schools, but there was little encouragement for the submission of broader program/study proposals. It should be noted, however, that at least one application for support of a Center for the Study of Medical Education was given extensive review and intensive discussion before being ruled outside the NSF mission.

For a new discipline seeking to establish itself, these rebuffs were undeniably discouraging. Although they did not deter continuing explorations and discussions with units of national government, they did stimulate the pursuit of alternative funding sources. One of these proved to be both substantive and catalytic in its contribution.

Between 1959 and 1961 the Committee on Professional Education of the American Heart Association was chaired by Stewart Wolf, a man with boundless energy and no perceptible limit in his willingness to explore unorthodox solutions to perplexing problems. Under his leadership a group of consultants laid the groundwork for a 1961 report called "The Physician's Continuing Education," to which reference has already been made (see Chapter 6). Among the concrete recommendations in this document were two describing specific educational research projects to be undertaken by the American Heart Association, and a third acknowledging the great need for experts in research in medical education that must be met if such projects were ever to be brought to fulfillment. The AHA Board of Directors must have been persuaded by these arguments, for the following year a budgetary line item led to the appearance of this announcement in *Circulation:*

> The American Heart Association recognizing the need for skilled personnel to guide professional education at undergraduate and postgraduate levels alike, has established a Fellowship Program to encourage interested basic or clinical scientists to embark upon the study of educational principles and methods of educational research.
>
> Candidates selected will be given an opportunity to receive training at one of the three medical schools that have established departments of research in medical education and to take part in the investigative programs in which these departments are engaged. They will also participate in the experimental pilot projects in continuing education now being established by the American Heart Association.

An accompanying commentary noted that "the Award was established to stimulate careers in the study of medical education and to prepare qualified physicians for leadership in this field." It is worth noting that four of the first six Fellows, all of whom elected to take their training at the University of Illinois Office of Research in Medical Education, have established themselves in positions that certainly represent fulfillment of this purpose: John Williamson, in the

School of Public Health at the Johns Hopkins University in Balti-
more; Clement Brown, now based at the South Chicago Community
Hospital; Alexander Anderson, in the Department of Medicine at
the University of Hawaii Medical School in Honolulu; and Joseph
Gonnella, associate dean and director of the Office of Research in
Medical Education at the Jefferson Medical College in Philadelphia.

Although the American Heart Association Fellowship was for several years the only general source of support for physicians seeking
further training in education, one other program, established in
1963, also highlighted the importance of preparing medically qualified personnel for their teaching responsibilities. The Milbank Faculty Fellowship set forth as the first two of six central objectives: (1)
to support accelerated career development for promising young faculty members, especially in their role as teachers; and (2) to improve
teaching skills and abilities, including the ability and willingness to
innovate in medical education and the ability to evaluate teaching.
Although this program was restricted to those following a career in
social and preventive medicine and provided no systematic interaction with educational scientists, it was nonetheless another manifestation of the emerging recognition that training in a specific
medical discipline was not enough to prepare faculty members for
their function as educators.

The second element of the American Heart Association support
program was an equally important demonstration. Initiation of
educational research pilot projects in three widely separated geographic areas, on both coasts and in a central Ohio community, had
symbolic as well as substantive significance. These projects, like the
first training programs, were also carried out in collaboration with
the Illinois ORME group.

The central Ohio study[1] was designed to document the acquisition and retention of new auscultatory skill by practitioners who
were exposed to intensive didactic instruction reinforced by heart
sound recordings, and the extent to which whatever new competence they acquired was translated into improved reporting of car-
diac sounds on the clinical records of their hospitalized patients. Although most participants improved their discriminatory skill, this
academic achievement was not reflected in hospital charts. Moreover,the skill that was gained suffered rapid decay. Distressing as
these findings may have been, they were perhaps less important
than the demonstration that careful study of the behavioral out-

come of continuing education programs was both possible and practical.

The East Coast/West Coast study, which took place in nine community hospitals, compared conventional lecture/conference instruction about selected cardiovascular diseases with consecutive case conference study of the same disorders.[2] The evaluation instrument in this instance was an early version of the patient management problem. This work led to further refinement in the design, use, and scoring of a tool that has now become a widely employed educational testing device.

The immediate impact of these studies may have been limited, but the example provided by the American Heart Association was of great importance. Although it did not trigger an avalanche of interest in supporting educational research and training by other voluntary health organizations, at the very least it heightened general awareness of the potential significance of these efforts.

It was certainly this general climate of growing interest in the systematic study of educational efficiency and effectiveness in medicine, coupled with the accelerating appeal of innovative instructional technology, that finally opened the door in Bethesda. Programmed instruction and teaching machines were among the most promising new devices on the educational horizon as the decade of the sixties began. These devices were being developed, refined, employed, and assessed, mostly at the elementary and secondary school levels although penetration of the collegiate setting was also beginning. The linear programming format, which was most widely used, seemed to have limited utility in teaching the basic and clinical sciences of medicine, where critical analysis and problem solving more than simple acquisition of information are major objectives. However, the more complex branched form, with optional pathways and remedial cycles, seemed to be readily adaptable to the content and goals of these disciplines. Seeing an opportunity, the Illinois group grasped it through an ambitious proposal for an interinstitutional study of this new automated teaching method.

In each of two years the project called for development and assessment of a two-week instructional unit in a basic science and a clinical subject comparing conventional lecture, programmed text, and teaching machine. Learning effectiveness was to be assessed by achievement tests designed to probe problem solving as well as information recall; learning efficiency was to be evaluated by a combination of achievement test scores and student study time data. In one of the experiments a conventional text was included as an instructional variable, and the differential costs of the four instructional modes were also to be compared in that study. When this proposal was submitted to the National Institute of General Medical Science it produced an encouraging initial response; subsequent notification that a two-year research grant had been both approved and funded was received with a sense of triumph.

But educational research, like the more familiar biomedical study, is not without unanticipated obstacles. Nearly four years were required to complete what had been projected for half that time. When it was done, the findings suggested that a teaching machine, although initially appealing, lost its charm rather quickly and offered no instructional advantage over a programmed text, which was far more portable and required no large investment in equipment. The study also revealed that the programmed form of instruction (whether delivered by book or machine) was in no instance more effective, and in only one instance more efficient, than conventional methods. The cost of preparing the programmed forms, either in money or in man hours, was so much greater than that of more familiar instructional devices that the question of justification for such an expenditure could not be avoided.[3]

Whether it was the disappointing outcome of this educational research and development project, the frustrating delays caused by technical problems of a kind unfamiliar to an institute staff accustomed to dealing with basic biomedical sciences, or changing program priorities, the hope that this work would lead to further support from the National Institute of General Medical Science did not immediately materialize. Despite the genuine interest of a sympathetic Institute director, further discussions about the development of basic science teacher training programs, and evaluation of the research training programs already in place, slowly withered and ultimately died.

By this time at least one other unit of the U.S. Public Health Service was beginning to evidence interest in exploring the potential applications of educational science to the improvement of health services through enhanced programs of continuing education. While he was an American Heart Association Fellow at ORME, John Williamson had been given responsibility for the initial phase of a medical school/community hospital collaboration in continuing education. The project was designed to provide an objective diagnosis of some educational need within the Rockford (Illinois) Memorial Hospital staff, the formulation of an educational prescription to meet that need, and an assessment of whether administration of specific educational therapy was successful in correcting the diagnosed deficiency. Although a familiar technique now, such an approach was novel then, and the Rockford laboratory data study has achieved almost classic status in the history of continuing medical education.[4]

Staff members of the Bureau of State Services (Community Health) had become interested in this methodology and encouraged ORME to develop a research grant proposal to extend the work. Although the resulting application, for support of "Educational Innovation to Improve Patient Care," was disapproved by the National Advisory Council, another branch of the Bureau picked up the idea as being consistent with the responsibility just assigned for implementing an entirely new federal initiative in continuing medical education, one that was not linked to disease categories (for example, neurologic disease and blindness), age groups (for example, child health), or specific interventions (for example, vocational rehabilitation). Following appropriate alterations of project scope, and the inevitable negotiations with fiscal officers, a one-year contract was awarded on April 1, 1965 for an initial phase of the work. It was labeled "Development of a System for Determining Priorities for Programs in Continuing Education." The project officer for this contract was Cecilia Conrath, whose supportive role over the next decade was of incalculable importance.

While these discussions and negotiations were taking place, the Bureau appointed a special committee on Health Education and Communication that provided an additional forum for the exploration of these ideas. The committee was charged to:

1. Review research and training practices in health education and communication, and activities in continuing education currently being conducted by Community Health divisions;
2. make an objective report of its assessment of programs as observed at the present time;
3. recommend goals and priorities, expansion or redirection of existing programs, new activities, and change in organization and staffing which it considers essential to keep abreast

of knowledge and technology in the field and to maximize the program effectiveness.

Through general meetings and special topic panel conferences, committee deliberations continued from October 1964 until November 1965. The final report appeared in February 1966. Among the thirteen specific recommendations it contained, only one is particularly significant in this narrative: "That the Public Health Service develop in institutions of higher learning and other continuing education facilities, regional demonstration centers for the purpose of training the teachers of the health professions in the effective use of educational science."[5] Although this statement was no more than a recommendation by a group of consultants who had neither authority nor control of purse strings, nonetheless it was a significant milestone on the path toward making educational research and development for the health professions not only visible but also viable. Since Bureau of State Services staff members (including Cecilia Conrath) had participated in the deliberations that led to this recommendation, there was reason to believe that the agency might now be ready to act within the limits of already established program guidelines and authorizations. This possibility took on the appearance of probability as the Illinois investigators, whose work on determining educational priorities was supported under a one-year contract, negotiated with federal sponsors a contract extension that incorporated this new program direction.

An agreement was consummated later in 1966 when a new contract was awarded for the first two years of a project that had as its ultimate goal the creation of a long-term demonstration center of continuing medical education. The funded Phase I included seven objectives: (1) formulation of a plan to develop a continuing education center for health personnel; (2) evaluation of the effectiveness and efficiency of the system for setting priorities in continuing medical education that had been developed under the original contract; (3) adaptation of the priority-setting system developed in a hospital setting for use in planning continuing education related to the care of ambulatory patients; (4) establishment of study groups in dentistry, nursing, and paramedical professions to develop long-range continuing education programs for different health professionals; (5) development of demonstration instructional programs to meet some of the additional continuing education needs now identified for physicians in Rockford; (6) evaluation of selected new and conventional methods of continuing education then being used; (7) design and implementation of pilot training activities for physicians responsible for conducting medical education programs.

The machinery was now in motion for a national program that could establish a precedent for funding health professions educational research and development, to match the well-established patterns for biomedical research and development through the National Institutes of Health and for general education research and development through the Office of Education.

Other potential sources of federal support outside the Public Health Service were not being neglected, however. Stephen Abrahamson, whose credentials were more familiar (and probably more highly regarded) than those of maverick educators from medicine, broke the barrier at the U.S. Office of Education. In 1965 that agency awarded his Division of Research in Medical Education at the University of Southern California two major grants. Both projects produced widespread repercussions among those interested in alternatives to conventional instructional modes.

The first study was carried out with the Department of Neurology, and more particularly with an imaginative neurologist named Howard Barrows. It had a two-part thrust, with each designed to improve the quality of learning how to perform a neurologic examination. The first component exploited the then new technology of cartridge-loaded single-concept films for mini-projectors. The product was a series of cartridges, with accompanying texts, that provided a remarkably complete self-instructional package.

Useful as this series proved to be, its impact was less significant than the "programmed patient," which was introduced, tested, and refined as the second element of this project. The idea of training a human model to simulate the historical features and physical manifestations of selected neurologic disorders was initially received with skepticism. However, the scoffers who later examined these programmed subjects soon discovered that the expected artificiality soon vanished as they became emotionally, as well as intellectually, captured by the remarkable reality of this simulated clinical encounter. An added dimension that simulation offered was the opportunity for direct, immediate, and standardized feedback from subject to examiner, not only about the degree to which critical findings were elicited but also about the subject's reaction to the historical inquiry and physical examination that had been carried out. Today the technique has been so refined and extended as to seem almost standard operating procedure in any first-rate clinical curriculum, but in 1965 it was not only novel, it was also daring.

The second project under Office of Education support was developed with J. S. Denson in the Department of Anesthesiology.[6] This too was a simulation, but of quite another kind. The mechanical/electronic marvel that emerged from the developmental work was called SIM I, and its features soon appeared in news media throughout the world. This computer-controlled model of a male body, lying on a standard operating table, responded to the administration of inhaled or intravenously introduced anesthetic agents, or other medications employed by anesthesiologists, with changes in blood pressure, pulse rate and volume, respiratory rate and depth, and pupillary size. It even produced the bucking movements that might accompany airway obstruction. Just as aircraft simulators allow pilots to learn their craft without endangering passengers, SIM I allowed anesthesiologists-in-training to administer potent anesthetic agents and to deal with emergencies that might arise during anesthesia without endangering patients. This simulation may still be the most sophisticated device yet introduced into the medical educator's armamentarium, although it now has a competitor developed by a group of cardiologists at the University of Miami.

Another source of support to which medical educators in general, and the growing group of educational research workers in particular, were now beginning to turn was industry. The National Fund for Medical Education had been created as a channel through which these organizations could funnel contributions without being subjected to repeated pleas from individual institutions or investigators. Directors of the fund welcomed applications for grants that would assist institutional efforts to strengthen medical education through systematic educational research and development. But more direct assistance was also forthcoming from specific industries when an educational research project matched their special interests or served their own needs. Abrahamson and Denson found this to be true when they approached the Aerojet General Corporation in connection with the development of SIM I. ORME at Illinois found a similar responsiveness in the International Business Machines Corporation when the idea of developing computerized patient management problems, in a natural language format, was proposed. In that instance IBM responded not only with the offer of terminal equipment and access to a giant computer in New York, but also with a grant-in-aid that permitted recruitment of some of the specialized personnel required for the work.

But it was not all peaches and cream. The bright promise of establishing national demonstration centers that was generated by the 1966 planning contract with the University of Illinois began to evaporate one year later when a reorganization of the U.S. Public Health Service caused the Bureau of State Services (Community Health) to disappear. Responsibility for further expansion of the work already under way fell to a new unit, the Bureau of Health Professions Education and Manpower Training, and a new project staff. Although this shift of responsibility did not diminish interest in the long-term project goals, it was not accompanied by the transfer of *contract* funds and authority that would allow the new agency to continue a program of the magnitude and duration conceived in the original discussions, and now detailed in the plan submitted as fulfillment of the first contract obligation. At most, the new bureau felt it could consider only relatively modest proposals, with any resulting contracts limited to one year. Thus the multiphase, long-term center concept was scuttled by an unexpected administrative and budgetary constraint.

Fortunately, research *grant* funds and authority did follow the transfer of responsibility, for otherwise the four-year Orthopaedic Training Study, initiated in 1964 (and ultimately extended through 1972), might also have come to a halt. This collaborative project between the Illinois Office of Research in Medical Education and the American Board of Orthopaedic Surgeons addressed basic questions of reliability and validity of the specialty board certification process, as well as the efficiency and economy of the specialty training experience.[7] Like an earlier study by the National Board of Medical Examiners, which aimed at more precise definition and assessment of clinical competence expected at the conclusion of internship, this work attempted to identify the critical components of competence required in the specialty practice of orthopaedics. The investigation went on to determine the extent to which the certifying examination methods then being used actually assessed these elements of performance; to develop new or refine old appraisal methods where discrepancies were found; to explore the pace at which these competencies were being achieved in approved residency training programs; to document the extent to which training experiences were designed to ensure acquisition of the required components of competence; and finally, to determine whether more efficient or more effective methods of learning these things might be devised and introduced into the training programs. This work proved to be a landmark study in graduate medical education and paved the way for subsequent investigations of a similar kind in pediatric cardiology (with the USC group), in child psychiatry (with the Illinois group), and in emergency medicine (with the Michigan State group), among others. But at this point in the story, the significance of the Orthopaedic Training Study lies in the fact that it was another milestone in the mobilization of support for educational research in medicine.

Comforting as it was to have, exciting as it may have been to implement, research and demonstration project support was not enough. If the work was to flourish, some way to support the training of those who would build upon this foundation also needed to be found. Helpful as they had been, the American Heart Association Fellowships alone could not meet the need, and the funding of teacher training programs by the Bureau of State Services had been brought to a halt after two promising years. As it turned out, the search for other alternatives ultimately led back once more to the National Institutes of Health.

In October 1965 President Johnson signed Public Law 89-239, the Heart Disease, Cancer, and Stroke Amendments of 1965. This legislation authorized a program of grants designed to encourage and assist in the establishment of cooperative arrangements among major health resources in discrete geographic regions still to be defined. The objective of the regional programs was to hasten the transfer of laboratory research findings about these categorical diseases into clinical practices that would benefit patients suffering from them. Administrative responsibility for implementing the legislative mandate was placed in the Office of the Director of the National Institutes of Health. Robert Marston, a well-known and widely respected academic administrator, was selected to head this new division. Marston was at the time dean of medicine and director of the Medical Center at the University of Mississippi, but he had formerly been an associate professor of medicine at the Medical College of Virginia and an enthusiastic participant in the 1960 AAMC/University of Illinois Summer Seminar on Medical Teaching. It was probably a significant indication of Marson's orientation when he included among a small group of advisors, assembled at Stone House in Bethesda a few months after his appointment, two individuals (Sanazaro and Miller) whose close identification with educational research and development was clear to all.

By mid-1966, this new program had achieved significant momentum. More than forty applications for planning grants had been received, and ten awards totaling more than $3,000,000 had been made. One common element running through both planning and operational proposals was probably stimulated by specific mention of continuing education in the authorizing legislation. This was not only an acknowledged area of need, if practitioners were to incorporate new knowledge into old practices, but also was one activity with which the applicants felt a comfortable familiarity—in contrast to the more amorphous functions embodied in the phrase "regional cooperative arrangements." But Marston had no intention of allowing the Regional Medical Program (RMP) to be used merely as a new way of supporting more of the same old thing; he saw it as an opportunity to transform and invigorate what had become a rather tired and conventional element of the educational continuum in medicine. The priority given to this thrust became evident when Marston plucked William Mayer from an associate deanship at the University of Missouri Medical School and installed him as the Associate Chief for Continuing Education in the Division of Regional Medical Programs. Shortly Mayer added two valued associates: Frank Husted, whose training in education began with Abrahamson at Buffalo and who was introduced to the health professions as director of the medical education unit at the Albany Medical College; and Cecilia Conrath, whose contribution to continuing education through the Bureau of State Services programs has already been noted.

In September 1966 the Division called together fifteen consultants, well known in continuing medical education, to give advice on a series of questions posed by staff about program direction and priorities. Among the things that emerged from this two-day conference was general agreement that a significant impediment to further development of new continuing education patterns and procedures was a shortage of professional personnel qualified to incorporate contemporary educational science into program planning and operation.

Such concurrence triggered acceleration of discussions on this question that had already been initiated with the University of Illinois Center for the Study of Medical Education (the outreach arm of ORME). By year's end, this unit had been awarded a one-year contract to set in motion an activity that could later be expanded and extended to other training sites as RMP operational issues and fiscal priorities were sorted out. By June 1967, the original contract to provide a one-year Fellowship in medical education for one physician/trainee and a 1-week seminar/workshop for 25 to 30 participants was expanded to an annual level of support for up to 12 trainees (now broadened to include other health professionals), two 3- to 6-week intensive introductions to educational science for 15 participants each, and four 1-week educational topic workshops, each to be offered to 25 health professionals who might contribute to the planning and implementation of RMP education and program evaluation efforts. At the University of Illinois, the work continued at this level until 1972, with some minor fluctuation in numbers from year to year. During that period, thirty-five Fellows spent at least one year in training (most earned an M.Ed. degree, four completed a Ph.D. in education); nearly 900 participants took part in workshops of 1 to 6 weeks' duration, while an additional 275 participated in more abbreviated workshops held in individual regions.

Illinois was not alone in this work, although it was the only unit with extensive and varied short-term program offerings both at the University and at regional sites. Within two years, contracts to establish Division of Regional Medical Program Fellowships had been negotiated with the medical education units at the University of Southern California, Michigan State, Ohio State, and the University of Washington. Together these schools produced another seventy-five graduates with at least one year of training in medical education. Unlike Illinois, whose trainees were almost entirely health professionals gaining experience and credentials in education, the other programs drew primarily from the discipline of professional education and were intended to introduce participants, through formal training, field experience, or both, to the special world of educational research and development in the health professions. It was fortunate that both populations were reached, for the work to be done could not be accomplished by either medicine or education alone. The bridging and linking functions that these trainees were able to fulfill, as they moved out into their professional assignments, seemed to lessen suspicion on one side and heighten pragmatism on the other.

For those most intimately involved in the promotion of educational research, development, and teacher training in the health professions, these were the lush years. Interest continued to grow, funds were more easily found, the battle for survival appeared to have been won, and a comfortable sense of security began to be felt. But we all knew the fragile nature of new federal bureaucracies, and the swiftness with which legislative interest and priorities can change. Thus it was not surprising when another reorganization of the Department of Health, Education, and Welfare shifted the Division of Regional Medical Programs out of NIH into a new Health Services and Mental Health Administration. Fortunately the program staff was essentially unchanged, and staff members remained supportive in their new establishment. True, Marston had been left behind as the new director of the National Institutes of Health, but his successor, Stanley Olson (once dean of the University of Illinois College of Medicine) was equally attuned to this educational need.

It was probably the change in signals coming from a new administration, coupled with congressional disillusionment about the cost-effectiveness of "regional cooperative arrangements" and competing demands for federal support in improving health services, that led first to funding constraints and finally to dismantling the entire Regional Medical Program. The training contracts were early victims of these forces; by 1972, all had been terminated. When this outcome seemed inevitable, a private appeal to Marston in his new role, late in 1971, gained a sympathetic ear; but other matters at NIH had higher priority and he was unable to provide any substantive response. His influence, however, must have been felt in the deliberations then under way in Congress.

As the decade of the seventies began, public concern for the physician shortage had reached such a peak that federal action to increase production of health manpower seemed essential. At the same time, the cost of medical education had risen to such a point that few private or public institutions felt able to increase class size without external assistance, and the cost of establishing new schools was thought to be beyond the resources of all but the most affluent public authorities or private benefactors. After extended and sometimes acrimonious debate, Congress intervened with Public Law 92-157, the Comprehensive Health Manpower Training Act of 1971.

In addition to providing general support, through capitation grants, to health professions schools that were prepared to respond with modest increases in class size, the legislation also provided authorization for special project grants that would allow fulfillment of special needs (for example, increased residency training in primary care, application of computer technology in health care demonstration programs). Among these special project categories was a provision for the establishment of grants to support training programs, traineeships, and fellowships, aimed at improving the teaching skills of established or potential health professions faculty members. It was a triumphant moment when the bill was signed, authorizing the appropriation of $10,000,000 for this faculty development purpose in fiscal year 1972, with $5,000,000 increments in each of the next two years. As usually happens in the two-stage congressional review and approval process, the subsequent appropriation was far less than the amount authorized. But at least it was the beginning of significant general support for health professions teacher training, support that did not have to be justified under a categorical disease label.

Most of the units that had mounted training programs under RMP contracts qualified for awards under the new legislation. It simply meant dealing with a new cast of characters in another federal agency, negotiating new agreements under somewhat different ground rules, using grant and contract rhetoric set to slightly different music. The important thing was that training program support now seemed assured, at least through the life of the original legislation. However, the congressional debate in 1974, when Public Law 92-157 came up for renewal, was very different from that which had taken place three years earlier. The major issues now were capitation itself and mechanisms for controlling both geographic and specialty distribution of physicians. These topics were so charged with implications and consequences that agreement on a new bill was delayed for two years. During that time continuing resolutions allowed many portions of the original act to proceed without interruption although with altered funding patterns. Unfortunately Section 769, which dealt with teacher training, was not among them. And when the new Health Professions Educational Assistance Act of 1976 emerged from Congress, Section 769 had been eliminated. It was a shattering blow, one with profound implications for the future of a movement that had now gained real momentum.

INTERNATIONAL REVERBERATIONS

8

During the midcentury decades the utility of educational research and development, and of teacher training, was increasingly recognized by North and South American medical educators, but this view was not generally shared by the worldwide community of their peers. In fact, on those rare occasions when that community assembled to exchange information and experience, the topic was more often received with apathy or even hostility than with interest or enthusiasm.

At the first such gathering—the 1953 World Conference on Medical Education held in London under the sponsorship of the World Medical Association, the World Health Organization, and the Council for International Organizations of the Medical Sciences—600 persons representing 127 faculties from 62 countries heard eighty-seven papers, of which only one directly addressed the question of preparing medical teachers for their educational responsibilities by design rather than by accident or incident. Even this presentation seemed to equate effective teaching with competence in lecturing. The remaining papers in the section of the meeting devoted to techniques and methods of medical education were little more than accounts of personal experience or illustrations of technical aids to instruction. There was virtually no reference to the data available even then on the conditions required to facilitate learning or to assess its achievement. Although a demonstration of audiovisual aids seemed to enchant the participants, the talk on training teachers was perhaps most widely received in the manner verbalized by one contributor: "How to teach? Teaching cannot be taught."[1]

By the time of the second world conference, held in Chicago in

1959, the University of Buffalo Project in Medical Education had flowered and the Association of American Medical Colleges had endorsed the ideas developed there, at least to the extent of jointly sponsoring two summer institutes on medical teaching. With Ward Darley's support, an effort was now made to interest the World Conference organizers in a similar seminar as a preconference or post-conference activity. The proposal produced no response beyond perfunctory acknowledgment. One section of the conference itself, however, was devoted to "the development of teachers and investigators." For those interested in the pedagogic component of this developmental process, it was disappointing that virtually all contributors focused their attention on the academic and disciplinary preparation of future faculty members, neglecting almost entirely their preparation as sound educators. In his conference summary comments, Dr. Donald Anderson, dean of the University of Rochester School of Medicine and one of the external reviewers of the Buffalo Project, observed that "medical schools have a responsibility to prepare prospective faculty members for their teaching responsibilities as well as for their roles as investigators . . . In the United States we have tended to put our trust in the view . . . that excellent teachers and leaders are always born from excellent investigators. As a result . . . in too many cases we find our faculties looking on teaching as only a sideline to their main activity—research. Of recent years, however, there has been increasing discussion of the possibility that a man's development as a teacher . . . should not be left to chance."[2]

This theme was echoed by more than a few of the other discussants of papers presented in this section of the conference. Among these contributors, I felt impelled to interject an observation that the time had come to replace expression of opinion about how medical education should be practiced with exchange of data, derived from research on learning and teaching, that could provide a more solid base for educational program planning and implementation.

Although a plea that the next world conference on medical education be organized around this theme failed to move the planners to do so, at least the 1966 meeting in New Delhi did include three working papers that addressed some of these issues, and several "fireside chats" (held under colorful tents) provided an opportunity to explore those questions further. In his concluding address, John Ellis commented on the welcome fact that since the first conference in 1953, "many lands and regions had founded associations for medical education, and older associations of medical schools have established sections for the study of the subject . . . Thus medical education in these years became a subject, lacking its own terminology but building a body of knowledge and expertise. In the forefront are those, few but increasing in number, and mainly American, who are devoting themselves to objective study and evaluation of teaching processes."[3]

By the time of the Fourth World Conference, held in Copenhagen in 1972, that number had multiplied manyfold. Several of those drawn from this new group even played a major role in planning, conducting, and evaluating the conference; the program itself included a full-day workshop devoted to teaching the teacher to teach. One reason for this growth in the international group of committed educational research and development experts was the conceptual and administrative encouragement given to such work by the World Health Organization (WHO) which, as Ellis noted in 1966, was becoming increasingly active in the field.

The preparation of teachers for schools of the health professions, particularly in the developing nations, has been a major concern of WHO since it was founded in 1948. During the early years program emphasis was understandably on providing opportunities for potential or established faculty members to expand their knowledge of biomedical sciences and of advanced techniques in medical diagnosis and treatment. Later this thrust was supplemented by efforts to deepen their understanding of such disciplines as preventive, social, and community medicine, which also addressed the organization and delivery of health care. Explicit organizational acknowledgment that preparation in subject matter is a necessary but insufficient qualification for the role of teacher first surfaced in a 1950 Expert Committee report. A section of this document dealing with instruction in teaching noted that "the Committee decided no general recommendations should be made. They did however recommend that instruction in teaching methods should be considered especially in underdeveloped areas where in new schools there was no body of teaching traditions."[4] A second report by the Expert Committee in 1952 did note that "In some places, junior faculty members from several institutions have been brought together and given a short training course in the art and science of 'education,' on an experimental basis. Although no definite conclusions can be drawn concerning the value of this procedure, there is considerable room for further experimentation of this kind."[5]

However, there is no suggestion in official records that anything was done to foster this experimentation at least until 1965, when another Expert Committee was convened to consider "The Training and Preparation of Teachers for Medical Schools with Special Regard to the Needs of Developing Countries." By this time medical education research and development practitioners in the United States had accumulated a decade of experience; the human relations in medical teaching program in Latin America was nearly five years old and had already involved more than 300 teachers in thirty-three countries; and the seeds for similar developments, which had been planted in other parts of the world, were in the process of germination. (For example, in Israel a Department of Medical Education had just been established at the Hadassah Medical School of Hebrew University under the direction of Dr. Moshe Prywes; and in the same year a program to improve teaching skills of medical faculty members had been initiated at the Central Institute for Advanced Medical Studies in Moscow.) Inevitably an Expert Committee that included among its members two leaders of such efforts (Prywes and Miller) would be influenced by their experience.

The committee report, however, went further than even these protagonists probably expected when the deliberations began. For the first time a significant segment of an official WHO document was devoted to elaboration of the importance of modern educational methods; of the need for research in educational processes to improve efficiency, effectiveness, and relevance of health professions education; and of the absolute necessity to provide more planned preparation in education for a much larger number of medical teachers. The recommendations with which the report concluded were clear and unequivocal:

1. The WHO Fellowship Program should be used to provide special opportunities for persons already qualified in a basic or clinical discipline to gain additional training in educational science. While most such WHO fellows would devote themselves to the acquisition of practical knowledge and skills, some should be encouraged to become proficient in educational research in medicine.

2. WHO should assist in the establishment of an international center or centers for training medical teachers in educational

science. Such centers should have a staff drawn from biological and educational sciences to mount continuing training activities of several types and of varied duration. They should serve as a professional resource to which educational institutions in medicine may turn for counsel, advice and assistance in the development of their own educational training activities or in the conduct of intensive self study.

3. The international center or centers described above should organize traveling seminars to bring expert help in education to individual institutions. Such a seminar might serve as a culminating event after a period of institutional self study.

4. Individual medical schools should be encouraged and assisted by WHO to establish within the framework of their own organizations, departments or divisions of medical education staffed by persons qualified to train medical teachers in the strategy and tactics of education as well as to coordinate the educational research upon which improved programs may be built.

5. WHO should encourage and assist in the support of educational demonstration programs in selected medical schools in developing countries that are prepared to explore new means of initiating first-rate medical education and that can be provided with staff who would assist them to engage in continuing investigations of the effectiveness of their programs, their methods, and their teachers. It is the belief of this committee that the present situation in respect to the training of medical teachers is so critical that the five proposals given above deserve prompt consideration and early implementation.[6]

But the wheels of a bureaucracy grind slowly. Two years later another Advisory Group, assembled in Geneva to evaluate the WHO program for education and training, noted once more:

The group believes that WHO should give much more emphasis to the training of teachers in the health and allied field. Alert to the principle of the "multiplier effect" of teacher-training, and aware that mere specialization and new acquisition of specialized knowledge do not necessarily produce teachers, the group recommends emphasis on a program of fellowships for *teachers,* not just specialists, to ensure an adequate flow of personnel for teaching institutions.

In addition to a knowledge of subject matter, teachers must know something about modern pedagogic methodology and the learning process, and have a grasp of the behavioral and ecological sciences. The last are important in placing medical and health practice in the proper community context.[7]

It is perhaps not surprising that these advisors expressed such an opinion, for the group included Moshe Prywes, whose contribution to this work has already been cited in several places; Alexander Robertson, who had organized the Saskatchewan teacher training effort (see Chapter 4) and was then director of the Milbank Memorial Fund, which had initiated an ambitious faculty development program; V. N. Butrov, from the Central Institute for Advanced Medical Studies in Moscow, whose teacher training efforts have also been noted; and Gabriel Velasquez Palau, a major figure in the Latin American effort to improve medical teaching.

During the next two years such activities accelerated, at least to the extent of introducing more teachers in health professions schools to the art and science of education. For example, the Pan American Health Organization program on human relations in medical education continued to spread across Latin American; a guidebook on the nature and uses of examinations in medical education was prepared by a group of WHO consultants and published as one of the Organization's Public Health Papers; the WHO European Office, in collaboration with the Scandinavian Federation of Medical Schools, organized a week-long workshop on examinations in medical education conducted at the University of Uppsala by consultants from the University of Illinois Center for the Study of Medical Education; the Southeast Asia regional office of WHO also invited the Illinois Center to conduct in New Delhi a four-week seminar in education for a group of medical teachers in that region. But most important in the development of a long-range program was the selection of teacher training as a major program priority in the Division of Education and Training at WHO Headquarters, and delegation of responsibility for this activity to a newly appointed Chief of Postgraduate Education.

Building upon what had gone before, Tamas Fulop began at once to mobilize the WHO resources required to establish a continuing and gradually expanding program that could ultimately embrace all member nations. One of his first actions, taken in November 1968, was to propose a "Consultation on the Organization and Program of Medical Schools Teacher Training" (later changed to ". . .

Program of Teacher Training for Health Personnel"), to advise on the form and content of such an effort. As one of the proposed participants, I was asked to assist with advance planning for this consultation. Out of these preliminary discussions came a working paper entitled "An International Program of Medical Teacher Training" that provided a framework for the subsequent deliberations and recommendations.

During the ensuing October 1969 meeting in Geneva, consultants* reviewed relevant documents, exchanged personal views, considered the contributions made by the WHO Headquarters secretariat and by advisors on education and training from three WHO regional offices, and heard the opinions expressed by representatives of other United Nations agencies. Out of these exchanges came a conclusion that "the problem of teacher training for the health professions is of such magnitude and of such central importance to the health of the world community that a systematic, sequential, worldwide attack must be launched without delay." But the consultants were also realistic enough to recognize that any implementation plan must ensure optimal utilization of scarce training resources; aim for the creation of a critical mass of trained personnel who could become self-sufficient first at a regional, later at a national, and finally at an institutional level; and employ a multiplier design rather than a linear or random action process.[8]

In order to achieve these goals, three levels of training were suggested. The first would be designed to produce *educational specialists,* either professional educators who would require familiarization with the realities, problems, and opportunities in health professions education, or those already qualified in a health profession who would need advanced training in education itself. At the second level the target would be *educational leaders,* health professionals who would acquire, through more abbreviated training, sufficient insight into educational science to foster its integration into the program planning, implementation, and evaluation activities of their own institutions. A third level would aim at *educational practitioners,* health professions teaching staff whose special training would be more limited and intended primarily to improve their competence as classroom, ward, clinic, or laboratory teachers.

---

*Drs. John Anderson and V. N. Butrov; Miss M. McIntyre; Drs. D. A. Messinezy, G. E. Miller, and V. Ramalingaswami.

With these purposes in mind, an organizational plan was proposed. It called for immediate designation of an Interregional Teacher Training Center (or Centers) devoted to the preparation of educational specialists, and of the educational leaders who could contribute to creating a receptive environment for the specialist's task of establishing Regional Teacher Training Centers (RTTC). These regional centers (the initial target was one in each of the six WHO regions) would in turn train the educational leaders who would organize National Teacher Training Centers (NTTC). The major task of national centers would be to increase the educational sophistication and competence of the classroom teachers who might later band together to create institutional units of medical education. This multiplier effect is illustrated diagramatically in Figure 8.1. The consultants anticipated that as more peripheral segments of the network gained strength and independent viability, the more central components would relinquish leadership and would serve increasingly in a responsive and supportive mode alone.

It is all very well to conceptualize a global program, but translating that conception into operational reality is quite another matter. That it was accomplished, and in a manner that closely resembled the initial plan, is a tribute to the ingenuity and vigor of Tamas Fulop, whose efforts to orchestrate the parts into a congenial whole began at once—and have never stopped. Even the most ingenious and creative international public servant recognizes, however, that the resolution of potential conflicts in the realm of autonomy/collaboration, dominance/subservience, and priorities/preferences among the proposed participants in such an enterprise takes time. In the meanwhile Fulop had another arrow in his quiver.

The World Health Organization has a well-established tradition of fostering linkages and encouraging exchange of information and personnel through the identification of special institutional resources whose contributions to global programs can be promoted by their designation as Collaborating Institutes. Before 1969 such centers had, with few exceptions, dealt with problems of disease surveillance, prevention, diagnosis, and treatment, or with specific areas of biomedical research. It was now proposed that two such units be nominated for their collaborative potential in medical education. Although this was an unusual suggestion, the growing worldwide importance of sharing educational research and development was becoming sufficiently well recognized to justify such a novel path.

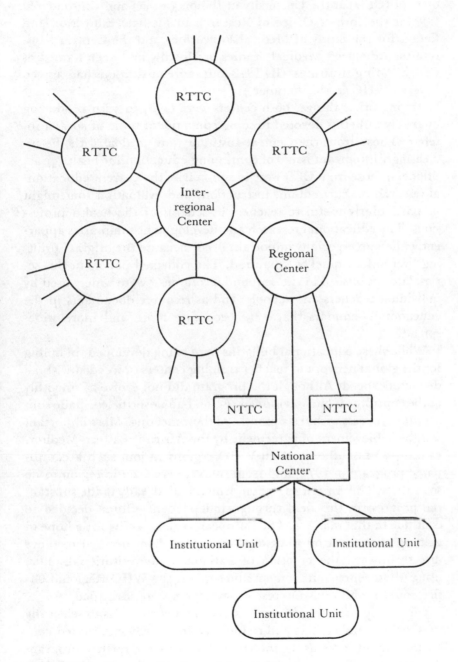

FIGURE 8.1. Network of teacher training centers.

By the last quarter of 1969, both the Center for Educational Development (CED) at the University of Illinois (a new and consolidated title for the former Office of Research in Medical Education and Center for the Study of Medical Education) and the Central Institute for Advanced Medical Studies in Moscow had been named as Collaborating Institutes. (By 1978 four more institutions had agreed to serve WHO in this manner.)

Among other things, both centers were charged with producing quarterly bulletins devoted to some educational topic of special interest. Those from the Central Institute were to deal with the increasingly important issues of continuing education for health practitioners; those from CED were to summarize the current educational research on curriculum, instruction, and evaluation that might be particularly useful to teachers in schools of the health professions. The educational research and development summaries apparently filled an especially important need, because the original printings were often quickly exhausted. The collected papers in this series, later published in two sequential volumes,[9] were widely used by individual teachers and schools, and as resource documents in the educational seminars that were becoming more and more widespread.

While these educational bulletins were being developed, planning for the global network of teacher training centers proceeded with all deliberate speed. Although the program did not evolve as smoothly as the consultants had envisioned, Fulop had nevertheless made substantial progress within six months of their meeting. Most important was the achievement of agreement by the African, Eastern Mediterranean, and Southeast Asian WHO regions to join such a coordinated program in 1971, and from the Western Pacific region to do so in 1972. The American region, which had already made substantial progress in this field through independent efforts, decided to continue in that manner. The European region, seeing little hope of gaining agreement on a regional center location, decided to move directly toward the creation of national and institutional units, using whatever encouragement and support the WHO Regional Office could mobilize as interested developers were identified.

One of the first tasks in establishing the network was to select the sites for regional centers and to identify an already established center that could serve as an interregional focus for further program development. The requirements for both types of centers had been set forth in general terms by the consultants (they are summarized in Table 8.1). Initially WHO was reluctant to establish the interregional center in a technologically advanced country, but in the face of such criteria there was little choice. After a period of cautious negotiation, the World Health Organization and the University of Illinois reached a formal agreement that the Center for Educational Development would provide the following programs in each of the academic years 1970-71 through 1973-74: (1) a one-year graduate-level program in health professions education for two to four candi-

TABLE 8.1. Criteria for Identification of Training Centers

The Interregional Center(s) should be established in an institution already identified as having acquired large experience in training teachers for the health professions. Such a center should satisfy the following criteria:

1. a sound record of producing teaching personnel of high quality;

2. an enviable reputation, as assessed by highly qualified educators in the health professions;

3. a wide scope of educational research and development activities, both in the institution itself and in the immediate academic environment;

4. a reputation for leadership in educational work, as well as the willingness, capacity, and experience to accept and train students at advanced levels;

5. evidence of strength and continuity of working relationships with other agencies;

6. a demonstrated willingness and capacity to serve as an international center for advanced training in educational science for the health fields;

7. such minimum institutional resources as full-time appointment of key staff; laboratories equipped for educational work; adequate library facilities; and financial resources sufficient for the maintenance, expansion, and renewal of all basic equipment;

8. the nucleus of full-time professional staff should include individuals specialized in such areas as (a) educational psychology, (b) educational sociology, (c) educational management, (d) curriculum evaluation and methods of measurement, (e) instructional methods; and additional supporting personnel.

For regional centers the criteria would be less strict but nevertheless of the same general character. The primary educational personnel of these centers may be part-time, initially, and may even come from other cooperating institutions. However, a minimum of one full-time staff member, preferably a generalist in education, would be required.

---

dates proposed by the Organization; (2) one 4-week seminar/workshop in Chicago for twelve to fourteen persons from the participating regions; and (3) one 2- to 4-week workshop for twenty-five participants at the site of an established or potential regional center. Through these three kinds of offerings it was expected that the interregional unit could, in the course of five years, train a cadre of educational specialists to serve as leaders for the regional programs, and contribute to the preparation and receptivity of regional institutions for the comparable work regional centers could carry out in developing national and institutional sites for further extension of the program.

Regional centers seemed to be the critical link in this chain, and more detailed guidelines were prepared to assist regional authorities in site selection. They included not only a set of primary and secondary factors that should be considered (such as willingness of administration and faculty to accept this responsibility, evidence of established commitment to excellence in training programs, and reflection of a multidisciplinary approach to health service delivery in the preparation of health professionals), but also the nature of support a host institution should be prepared to commit to the proposed regional center (for example, assurance that the RTTC would function as a department with the same academic standing as other departments; the provision of space and basic support personal). The regional centers were not seen as WHO appendages to a university, but as integral units of a university that might receive assistance from WHO in the form of fellowships for staff, tuition payments for long- and short-term trainees accepted by the center, and even limited support for equipment and supplies. Since the quality of staff and trainees was a vital ingredient in these programs, a set of suggestions for consideration in selecting such personnel was also developed.

With these preparatory tasks completed, the work of the program itself began. However, the practical implementation of a complex enterprise involving groups that are widely separated geographically, culturally, and administratively is inevitably more difficult than a neat planning document might suggest. This program, with principal bases in Geneva, Chicago, Brazzaville, Alexandria, New Delhi, and Manila, was no exception to that general rule. Regions were at different stages in their readiness to undertake teacher training activities; communication channels sometimes seemed tortuous and unresponsive; ambiguities in definition of responsibility and authority appeared in unexpected ways; different interpretations of what was meant by "advance planning" often abraded otherwise smooth tempers; and individual preferences in program focus or emphasis were occasionally at odds with the pattern established by those responsible for coordination. Nonetheless, the 1972-73 interval was a period of remarkable progress.

Initially the African region was the most enterprising in launching the work. Even before the final accord had been signed or regional sites selected, a regional workshop was organized with assistance from the Interregional Center, and two candidates were proposed for the master's degree program in 1970. Within the next year Regional Office staff identified Makerere University in Kampala, Uganda, as the site for an English-language regional center, and the University Center for the Health Sciences in Yaoundé, Cameroon, as the setting for a French-language center. In subsequent years the director-designate from each took part in the master's program at Illinois.

In 1971 the Eastern Mediterranean Regional Office asked consultants from WHO Headquarters and the Interregional Center to visit and assess the qualification of an institution that had tentatively been selected as the regional center site. Their recommendation led to negotiations that resulted in the designation in 1972 of Pahlavi University School of Medicine in Shiraz, Iran (now the University of Shiraz) as the regional center. Anticipating that outcome, by the end of 1971 the director-designate was enrolled in the CED master's program, and ten members of the Pahlavi Medical School faculty had taken part in a short-term workshop in Chicago. Seven more participated in a 1972 on-site workshop in Shiraz.

In April 1971 a similar team was asked by the Western Pacific Regional Office to visit Sydney, Australia, for comparable review of a potential regional site there. Establishment of the regional center at the University of New South Wales was recommended by the consultants, but lengthy negotiations among the Regional Office, the University, and the Australian government delayed formal implementation until 1973. By that time, however, twelve members of the medical faculty had taken part in short-term programs at the University of Illinois and seventeen more had participated in an on-site workshop. The first director of the regional center had just completed service as dean of the New South Wales Faculty of Medicine; his successor in the directorship later won a master's degree in education at the Michigan State University Office of Medical Education Research and Development.

During November and December of 1971, a single consultant visited both Thailand and Sri Lanka at the request of the Southeast Asia Regional Office. Before that year ended two regional centers had been designated: one at the University of Sri Lanka in Peradeniya, the other at Chulalongkorn University in Bangkok. The director-designate of each center earned a master's degree in education at the University of Illinois; a second staff member from each center later completed a similar program of study at CED; and a third from each did so at the University of Southern California Division of Research in Medical Education. In addition, seven faculty members from Chulalongkorn later came to Chicago for a short-term program, and nine more participated in an on-site workshop in Bangkok. At Peradeniya no on-site workshop was conducted by the Interregional Center, but two were independently organized and conducted with the assistance of consultants from the University of Southern California group. Only two members of the Peradeniya faculty participated in short-term programs in Chicago.

Another activity that was not included in the original master plan, but which represented an important addition to the overall program, was a special interregional workshop held in Chicago in 1971. It was designed for selected national and institutional leaders who would not themselves be involved in the operation of regional centers but whose understanding and support were essential if the overall plan was to succeed. A similar workshop for French-speaking leaders was conducted by WHO headquarters staff members in Yaoundé, Cameroon, the following year.

By 1972 the first phase of this ambitious effort to launch a coordinated worldwide program of health professions teacher training was drawing to a close. The stage had been set in 1965; a specific plan had been elaborated in 1969; and in the short space of three years a vigorous program had taken form. It was now time to review what had been accomplished and to suggest the next steps, if in fact next steps were desirable.

The study group that was assembled in October 1972 at WHO headquarters in Geneva included two members of the 1965 Expert Committee, one who had served in the 1967 advisory group, two who had taken part in the 1969 consultation, and three regional teacher training center directors, as well as Division of Education and Training staff members who had been responsible for operational planning and supervision of the program. The tone of the meeting was clearly different from that of the earlier gatherings. The accelerating pace of health professions educational research, development, and teacher training had produced a more sophisticated panel of contributors as well as the establishment of more widely dispersed support resources. There was also a changing mood both within and outside WHO about the desirability, even the propriety, of a centrally directed program of this kind. The shift was not reflected in any disagreement about the continuing need for vastly increased numbers of health professions teachers trained in the science of education, but in an undercurrent of uneasiness about the organizational structure that had been designed to encourage achievement of that goal. In fact, a March 1972 editorial in the *British Journal of Medical Educaton* went so far as to comment: "The principles of good higher education may be the same the world over, but it may well be that their successful application will depend on careful attention to local conditions. Indeed it may not be altogether wise to assume that the principles themselves are all known or fully understood anywhere. The World Health Organization pyramidal structure for medical teacher training is not without its dangers."

The program had not, of course, been visualized by the initial planners as pyramidal, with truth flowing down from apex to base; it had been pictured as ever-widening concentric circles of activity, much like those generated when a stone is dropped into a quiet pool with the central agitation disappearing as the waves move outward. Nonetheless, Regional Offices were beginning to feel constrained by a structure that did not always seem optimally responsive to their interests, their budgetary limitations, and their timing. With a growing number of institutions now prepared to offer teacher training opportunities, it was understandable that they might seek alternative pathways.

After four days of discussion and debate, the study group endorsed the general purpose of the initial program and applauded the progress that had been made. They then went on to say:

> In carrying out the program outlined in the 1969 report, attention was first given to the principle of establishing a critical

mass of concerned and informed individuals initially at regional sites, then providing for continuity of relationship between interregional, regional and national groups while working toward the growing independence of all. The momentum
achieved suggests that additional principles can now be incorporated in further program implementation: (i) while central
coordination of such a program will remain important, the
principle of greater flexibility and diversity at regional and local levels will contribute to furthering the development of the
program; (ii) the principle of greater support for local and national centres/units to develop on their own will further the
program whether or not a regional center exists. The experience of certain countries illustrates the need to foster alternative strategies when circumstances delay the identification of a
regional center or when for other reasons it may seem undesir-
able.[10]

Although the words called for continuing central coordination
the spirit called for central cooperation but decentralized planning
and direction. In the light of progress this seemed a reasonable step.
In keeping with this spirit, the formal agreement with the University
of Illinois was allowed to lapse upon completion of the training commitments made for 1972-73. By that time, 13 Fellows had completed the one-year training programs, 54 had taken part in the
Chicago workshops, and nearly 100 had participated in regional
workshops conducted by the Interregional Center (a breakdown of
participants is shown in Tables 8.2 and 8.3). From this point on the
Center for Educational Development, like comparable units elsewhere, would respond only to specific institutional, national, or regional requests for assistance. Responsibility for more general plan-
nng and coordination would shift from a global Geneva/Chicago
axis to the more restricted geographic focus of WHO Regional Offices, where familiarity with local needs and required resources
would be more intimate. The ultimate goal, however, remained unchanged: the establishment by 1980 of a national teacher training
center in each member nation that wanted such a program. Before
the decade ended that goal was modified, but the story of that
change can be told later.

With adoption of this new orientation the work continued to thrive.
A comprehensive study of the program's progress and impact is now
being carried out by a group of consultants under the direction of

TABLE 8.2. Number of Participants, WHO Fellowships and Workshops, University of Illinois at the Medical Center, Center for Educational Development

Regions	Fellows			
	1970-71	1971-71	1972-73	1973-74
African	1	2	3	1
American	0	0	0	0
Eastern Mediterranean	0	1	0	1
European	0	1	0	0
Southeast Asian	1	1	1	0
Western Pacific	0	0	0	0
Total	2	5	4	2

Regions	Four-Week Workshops—Chicago			
	1971*	1972 (1)	1972 (2)	1973
African	1	0	1	0
American	2	2	0	0
Eastern Mediterranean	4	4	5	7
European	1	0	0	0
Southeast Asian	2	3	3	4
Western Pacific	2	4	5	4
Total	12	13	14	15

*Two-week program for selected leaders.

Dr. Fred Katz. However, illustrations of what has been occurring in each of the several world regions, both within and outside the WHO sphere of influence (at least up to the time of a review meeting in 1976), may help to round out the international picture.

The *African region* appears to have experienced the greatest difficulty in mounting a comprehensive program, although admittedly it has been more difficult to gain information about regional activities there than elsewhere. In 1976 each of the two regional centers was a one-man operation, with little evidence of integration into the life of either host institution. Without question the unsettled political situation in Uganda compromised the internal and external work of that regional center. And in Yaoundé, there was at least suggestive evidence that internal conflicts and competing priorities

TABLE 8.3. Number of Participants, WHO On-Site Workshops, University of Illinois at the Medical Center, Center for Educational Development

Region	Total Participants	Multiple Participants from One Country	Multiple Participants from One Institution
African			
Kampala 1970	24	5 Uganda	5 Makerere University
		5 Nigeria	4 Univ. of Nairobi
		4 Kenya	3 Univ. of Ibadan
		3 Ghana	3 Univ. of Ghana
		2 Zambia	2 Univ. Of Abidjan
		2 Ivory Coast	2 Univ. of Lagos
			2 Univ. of Zambia
Accra 1972	17	8 Ghana	8 Univ. of Ghana
		5 Nigeria	2 Univ. of Dar Es Salam
		2 Tanzania	
Eastern Mediterranean			
Shiraz 1972	20	11 Iran	7 Pahlavi Univ.
		2 Egypt	2 Univ. Of Isfahan
			2 Univ. of Alexandria
Shiraz 1973	16	7 Iran	4 Pahlavi Univ.
		3 Egypt	2 Univ. of Alexandria
		2 Ethiopia	2 Univ. of Addis Ababa
		2 Sudan	2 Univ. of Khartoum
Southeast Asian			
Bangkok 1972	25	19 Thailand	9 Chulalongkorn Univ.
		6 Indonesia	3 Ramathibodi Univ.
			3 Sirriraj Univ.
			3 Chiangmai Univ.
			2 Univ. of Indonesia
Western Pacific			
Sydney 1971	23	20 Australia	17 Univ. of New South Wales

had blunted the thrust of both the institutional and regional programs.

In the *American region,* on the other hand, the most expansive, comprehensive, and well-supported of all the regional centers is still functioning at the Federal University of Rio de Janeiro. The program there is jointly sponsored by the University, the federal government, and the Pan American Health Organization (PAHO). Between 1973 and 1976 the center conducted fifty workshops, in which more than 800 representatives of all the major health professions participated (some 400 of the participants came from the host university). The center operates with a professional and technical staff of nearly 50 persons, on an annual budget in excess of $800,000. Because the center was designated as one of two PAHO-supported Latin American Centers for Educational Technology for Health (CLATES), an early program emphasis was the utilization of technical aids to education such as television, film, audio-cassettes, and computers as instructional alternatives. However, the elaboration of instructional materials and curriculum patterns appropriate to less affluent sectors of the region was also given due attention.

The second CLATES, in Mexico City, had also directed major attention to the optimal development and utilization of technology. Unfortunately, changing leadership resulted in far less visible program implementation, but there appeared to be little question that the work had influenced substantial numbers of Mexican medical teachers, even though detailed documentation of progress was more difficult to find.

With the assistance of these central facilities, the Pan American Health Organization proceeded to establish an extended network of secondary units in medical, dental, and nursing schools throughout the Latin American community. Each is known as a Nucleus for Educational Technology for Health (NUTES).

The *Eastern Mediterranean Region Center,* which also functions as the Department of Medical Education in Pahlavi University Medical School, has had a remarkable impact on the region as well as on the host institution. In the period from 1972 to 1975, the center offered thirty-nine workshops; sixteen of these were for individual schools within the region and twelve were for national groups outside Iran. A consistent theme in this work was the exposition of a systems approach to educational planning, with practical demonstrations of how it could be applied. Some 660 faculty members from twenty institutions were included in these programs, and a residual "cell" of educational research and development activists can now be identified in at least ten of those schools. Virtually all the participants came from medical schools; involvement of other health professions has been very limited.

Although the impact of these activities has probably been least felt in Iranian medical schools in general, this observation would not hold true for the host institution. At Pahlavi University a relatively small permanent staff has clearly influenced curriculum organization (including the development of a new, community-based, second medical school), instructional methods, and the student evaluation system.

Activities in the *European region* are most difficult to capture in a summary paragraph, since there has been no regional center to serve as a focal point for these efforts. Yet in nearly every European country, eastern as well as western, some significant health professions educational research and development group can be identified. Among the most prominent units would certainly be that at the University of Bern; the Center for Medical Education in Dundee, Scotland; the medical education staff at the University of Limburg Medical School in Maastricht, the Netherlands; the Department of Educational Research and Development at the Medical Center for Postgraduate Education in Warsaw; the British Life Assurance Trust Center for Health and Medical Education in London; and the Faculty of Medical Education in the Central Institute for Postgraduate Studies in Moscow. In addition, there must be dozens of smaller official units, or functional groups without official designation, that add to regional vigor in this field.

It is worth noting that the first major international investigation of medical student achievement in different educational systems was initiated in the European region. Organized by Hannes Kapuste in Germany, the Tripod Study included Jean-Jacques Guilbert in France and Christine McGuire in the United States as principal collaborators, This effort was also an important stimulus to the formation of a regrettably short-lived International Association for Research in Medical Education (IRME).

In *Southeast Asia,* with two regional centers, there has been relatively little coordinated regional activity, although each of the centers has had a perceptible influence on educational program development in the host school or nation. From 1971 to 1975, the group in Peradeniya had organized sixteen workshops that reached 230 individual participants, of which roughly 20 percent came from faculties other than medicine. The impact of this work was most evident in the parent medical school, although some limited effect appears to have been felt by several other health professions educational programs within Sri Lanka. A general university requirement that all faculty members have some training in education has led to the assignment of this responsibility in the health fields to the Peradeniya Center.

The Chulalongkorn center in Bangkok has devoted itself largely to establishing a mutual support network of educational research and development interests among the health professions schools in Thailand. The attempt to organize a national consortium as a substitute for the single institutional concept of a national center was an interesting variant on the basic theme, but it appears to have had limited success. Nevertheless, by 1976 the Bangkok unit involved more than 650 people, drawn from both health professions education and the health service delivery systems, in training activities of varying kind and duration.

The *Western Pacific Regional Center* in Sydney is also the Center for Medical Education at the University of New South Wales. Like CLATES-RIO, it has drawn support from multiple sources, including the University, the federal government, WHO, the United Nations Development Program (UNDP), and the Kellogg Foundation, among others. The Sydney Center has perhaps the most fully developed system for matching training programs with the identified needs of a regional constituency, and for follow-up to assess outcome as well as to ensure continuing assistance if it is required. By 1976, the regional center staff had conducted some forty workshops of various kinds for a variety of health personnel institutions (including those devoted to training nonprofessional primary care providers in Fiji and in Papua New Guinea), government health agencies, and professional organizations. The University of New South Wales unit also has a well-organized master's degree program in health professions education, which is individually tailored to prepare participants for the role to which they will return. An important feature of the program is the action research project that all candidates must carry out in the home institution.

The major work of implementing the global program that kindled worldwide interest in health professions educational research, development, and teacher training has unquestionably been carried out in many widely separated sites. Nonetheless, it is also important to note the continuing substantive and catalytic contributions of staff members in the WHO Headquarters Division of Health Manpower

Development (successor to the Division of Education and Training). This unit is now headed by Tamas Fulop, the original driving force for the comprehensive, sequential worldwide program.

In the conduct of teacher training workshops, Jean-Jacques Guilbert (Chief Medical Officer for Educational Planning), a physician who won his doctorate in education at the University of Southern California Division of Research in Medical Education, is almost without peer. Guilbert has both refined the workshop format through repeated use (personally conducting five to eight such programs each year) and created an educational handbook designed to serve as a centerpiece for the individual and small-group study that now characterizes most of his workshop offerings. Available in English, French, Bulgarian, Czech, German, Hungarian, Italian, Polish, Portuguese, Russian, and Spanish, the handbook is a remarkable basic reference, imaginatively set up to capture attention and to assure active reader involvement without sacrifice of substance.

At a time when audiovisual technology was spreading unrestrained and weed-like through the health professions education community, M. A. C. Dowling (Chief Medical Officer for Educational Communications Systems) attempted to bring some order out of that chaos. As the Division's educational communications specialist Dowling was beset by a continuing stream of visitors, each seeking advice on which of the dazzling instructional aids was best (often forgetting the electrical and mechanical maintenance requirements for many of them). Dowling assembled a comprehensive collection of hardware and software in a demonstration center that has proved invaluable. His own research and development interests have led him increasingly in the direction of finding or devising appropriate educational technology for emerging nations with limited resources, and developing accompanying software that is appropriate to the cultural standard and literacy level of the target population.

A central feature of the original teacher training program was to prepare teachers who would educate students to meet the real health needs of the settings in which they would work, using available health service resources. However, faculty members preoccupied with physician education (often aimed to meet "international standards") and with hospital care often overlooked the fact that in many countries a substantial amount of preventive as well as curative service is delivered by other health personnel in nonhospital settings. The role of such workers in the health service system, and their educational needs, are often neglected. Daniel Flahault (Chief Medical Officer for Health Team Development) is concerned primarily with this group of health care providers. His efforts have surely increased general awareness of the importance of these aides, auxiliaries, village health workers, and traditional birth attendants, and of the great need for instructional material suited to their background and functions.

The most recent addition to this headquarters group is a Chief Scientist for Educational Evaluation. Fred Katz was director of the Tertiary Education Research Center at the University of New South Wales and an important contributor to the development of the regional center there. Since his arrival in Geneva, Katz has been in constant demand as an advisor to other divisions responsible for mounting and evaluating training programs in the area of their special interests; to regional personnel who regularly seek better means of evaluating the education, training, and health service programs for which they are responsible; and to colleagues in the Division of Health Manpower Development as they formulate broad program initiatives that necessarily include an evaluation component.

In sum, progress on the international front of educational research and development for health has been substantial and continuing. Looking back over the years since 1956 it is difficult to believe that so much has been accomplished so quickly or that so many people have been caught up in the work. It is certainly a far cry from the apathy, or frank hostility, with which the science of education was regarded when these years began.

ASSIMILATION AND INTEGRATION

9

Now the web grows more tangled. It was relatively easy to tease apart the evolutionary threads when the work was closely identified with no more than a handful of individuals and institutions; by mid-1977, however, preliminary exploration revealed seventy-two medical schools in the United States and Canada that seemed to have a clearly established unit of educational research and development. Sixty-seven responded to my inquiry about organization, staffing, functions, and support; the data from sixty were sufficiently complete to justify inclusion in this summary of what was then the state of things.

The description given here represents at best a sketch rather than a definitive portrait—and it is subject to change without notice. Since the questionnaire was circulated, at least three more units have sprung up and at least one may have vanished. The numbers will probably have changed again by the time these words appear in print, but it is unlikely that the order of magnitude will be greatly different. For reference, Table 9.1 shows where then current programs were located and the year in which each was established.

The units do their work under a bewildering array of labels (Table 9.2). Only five are officially recognized as academic departments within the parent school (two carry departmental titles), although nearly a third report that they function as academic programs. The largest number describe themselves as professional resources without academic status; the remainder see themselves as professional/technical or simply as technical support services without academic recognition. Less than a third of the units can themselves award academic rank to professional staff. In most programs staff members have their academic appointments in well-estab-

TABLE 9.1. Medical Education Research and Development Units in the United States and Canada

Founding Date and Location	
1958 Western Reserve University	1972 University of Arizona
1959 University of Illinois	University of California at
Medical College of Virginia	San Francisco
1962 Albany Medical College	University of Iowa
1963 University of Southern	University of Kansas
California	McMaster University
University of Rochester	Meharry Medical College
1965 Medical College of Georgia	University of Minnesota
1966 Michigan State University	University of Nebraska
Ohio State University	Southern Illinois University
1967 University of Toronto	University of Utah
SUNY at Syracuse	1973 Laval University, Quebec
Temple University	University of New Mexico
Tufts University	Queens University, Ontario
University of Washington	University of Texas at
1968 University of Alabama	San Antonio
University of California at	George Washington University
Davis	1974 University of British Columbia
University of Colorado	Columbia University
University of Connecticut	McGill University
Georgetown University	University of Mississippi
University of Missouri	New Jersey Medical School
Wayne State University	Northwestern University
1969 University of Florida	University of Oregon
Jefferson Medical College	1975 Chicago Medical School
1970 University of Calgary	Hahnemann Medical College
University of Kentucky	Rush University
University of Nevada	Rutgers Medical School
University of North Carolina	University of South Dakota
University of Pittsburgh	1976 SUNY at Buffalo
University of Virginia	University of Pennsylvania
1971 University of Maryland	1977 Albert Einstein Medical School
University of Texas Medical	Medical University of South
Branch, Galveston	Carolina
University of Western Ontario	Medical College of Wisconsin
	1978 University of North Dakota

TABLE 9.2. Medical Education Unit Designations

Office of Medical Education   (11)
Office of Education   (4)
Division of Research in Medical Education   (3)
Office of Research in Medical Education   (2)
Office of Educational Resources   (2)
Center for Educational Development
Center for Medical Education
Department of Research in Health Education
Department of Health Sciences Education
Division of Educational Measurement and Research
Division of Educational Development
Division of Educational Planning and Assessment
Division of Educational Service and Research
Division of Educational Support and Development
Division of Learning Resources
Division of Medical Education and Communication
Division of Educational Communication
Division of Research and Evaluation in Medical Education
Division of Studies in Medical Education
Educational Resources Group
Educational Planning and Development Program
Learning Resources Unit
Medical Learning Resources
Office of Curricular Affairs
Office of Curriculum Affairs
Office of Curriculum Affairs and Education Resources
Office of Curriculum Development and Evaluation
Office of Educational Research
Office of Educational Research and Development
Office of Educational Research and Services
Office of Educational Resources and Research
Office of Educational Services
Office of Educational Sciences
Office of Health Sciences Education
Office of Medical Education Research and Development
Office of Medical Studies
Office of Research and Development in Medical Education
Office of Service and Research in Medical Education
Office of the Coordinator for Educational Development
Program for Educational Development
Research and Evaluation in Medical Education

lished, and presumably supportive, medical school departments (more commonly clinical than basic science), or occasionally in the faculty of education.

In keeping with the original concept that medicine and education were equal partners in this venture, three of the first six units were headed by physicians and three by professional educators. The subsequent trend, however, has tilted sharply toward the latter: forty-two of the sixty units responding are headed by persons whose basic professional identity is with education; only fourteen directors hold doctorates in medicine (six of these also have advanced degrees in education). It is striking to note, however, that three-fourths of these leaders, whether they were trained primarily in education or in medicine, have been in the field of *medical* education research and development for more than five years.

Among the fifty-one units that reported their position in the university organization, thirty-eight are in the college of medicine while thirteen are based in a health center. Directors of the former group generally report to the medical school dean (or, less frequently, to a senior associate in the dean's office), whereas the latter usually report to the vice president for health affairs or a deputy. Whether this proximity to the highest administrative officers represents, or is perceived as, a direct delegation of academic responsibility or simply suggests a technical service function to administration is not always clear.

The units range in size from two with no full-time professional or technical staff, to three with more than fifty; the mean figure is 10, the median and modal numbers are 5. Virtually all units offer professional assistance to faculty in the design and development of curriculum, instructional materials, and evaluation procedures, as well as in the improvement of teaching practices. Among the technical services proffered, those related to the administration, scoring, and reporting of examinations are almost universal. Some of the larger units also provide photography, television, and other audiovisual services; a few seem to do little else. Although a substantial majority of the units are engaged in educational research, thirteen report that this is not presently a part of their work.

The inquiry about faculty development, currently popular in higher education, produced more spontaneous comment than any other item in the questionnaire. Although eighteen respondents denied offering any formal program that would qualify under this heading, many coupled this negative response with the remark, sometimes barely concealing annoyance, that they regarded every encounter with faculty as part of an educational development effort. A number of those who did report such formal offerings made the same observation. So be it. However they were described, the activities labeled "faculty development" most often fell within the category of in-service training, presumably on-the-job developmental activities. Less than half of the units offered short-term (that is, lasting more than one day) educational programs; thirteen scheduled 1- to 6-month programs and nine listed 6- to 12-month training opportunities. Formal graduate programs were offered by nine units, but in only one was the medical education unit itself completely responsible; in the rest a collaborative program provided a major experience in health professions education, but much of the course work and the degree as well were given by the college of education.

The thirty-two units that responded to questions about the magnitude and source of support reported annual budgets ranging from $45,000 to $1,700,000, with a mean of $284,000. Although both the absolute amounts and the range are of interest, they should be considered as order of magnitude rather than as strictly comparable reports from institution to institution. For example, some units reported that they had no independent budget but were supported according to need and the availability of funds in the office of a dean or other administrator. Other respondents included program but not personnel budgets since these funds were derived through different channels. Some included income from technical services while others did not; some reported allocations from capitation grants as part of institutional funds while others listed them separately; a few gave only percentage distribution without absolute dollar figures while others gave both. Nevertheless, with all these reservations, the distribution data in Table 9.3 do offer some insight into funding patterns.

The picture that emerges is one of widespread activity that varies both in character and intensity from institution to institution. It is carried out under many administrative arrangements and with a wide range of staff and budgetary resources. There is no typical unit, nor is it possible to identify a model that has won general emulation. The nature of the organization and the work in any setting seems to reflect more the commitment of institutional leadership and the vigor of unit leadership than the adoption of any universal

TABLE 9.3. Medical Education Unit Budgets

Budget Elements	No. of Respondents	%	$ (in thousands)
Total			
Range	32	—	45-1,700
Average	—	—	284
Source			
Regular institutional			
appropriation — amount			
Range	28	—	19-937
Average	—	—	160
Regular institutional			
appropriation — % of total			
Range	40	13-100	—
Average	—	64	—
Capitation funds — amount			
Range	11	—	14-239
Average	—	—	80
Capitation funds — % of total			
Range	16	5-92	—
Average	—	39	—
Grants and Contracts — amount			
Range	22	—	4-1,400
Average	—	—	146
Grants and contracts — % of total			
Range	28	5-100	—
Average	—	29	—

body of principle and practice. Although there now seems to be general acceptance of the thesis that educational science does have something to contribute to the practice of medical education, the substance of that contribution, the personnel best able to provide it, and the organizational arrangement required to achieve it are as varied as the institutions that offer it.

Nevertheless, there are a few programs to which visitors from the United States and abroad seem to turn with some regularity as they look for working examples, if not models. Among the most prominent are those that have been identified for a decade as the big three: the Center for Educational Development (CED) at the University of Illinois at the Medical Center, the Division of Research in

Medical Education (DRME) at the University of Southern California, and the Office of Medical Education Research and Development (OMERAD) at Michigan State University. Perhaps one reason is the breadth of their seed sowing, illustrated in Figures 9.1, 9.2, and 9.3. These maps show only institutional sites where graduates or former staff members have been implanted as program directors. Impressive as such graphic representations may be, the criterion employed in their creation has simply assured a map of manageable dimensions, not one that conveys a full picture of the diffusion of personnel from any one of these units. For each center has produced many persons who, though not program directors, fill influential administrative positions in health professional schools, play important leadership roles in academic departments, or carry significant responsibility for educational development in national organizations. If all the long- and short-term trainees were also included, virtually every medical school in North America — and a substantial number in Western Europe, the Middle East, Africa, and the Far East — would also be listed.

This is not the place for a comprehensive description of these or other programs, nor is it possible to offer any comparative judgment of their worth or impact. Nonetheless, an elaboration of some of the similarities and differences between and among these most promi-

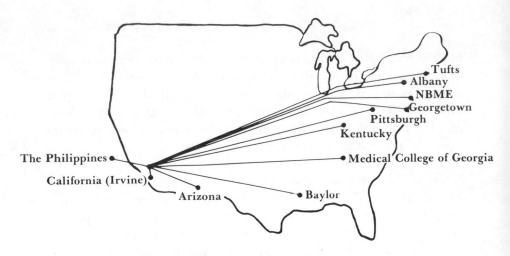

FIGURE 9.1. University of Southern California colonization.

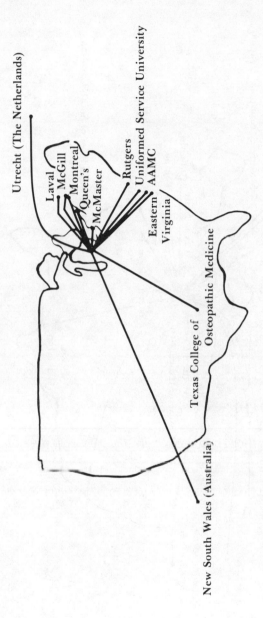

FIGURE 9.2. Michigan State University colonization.

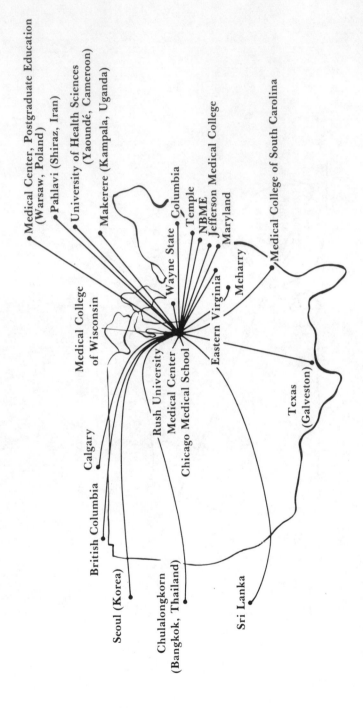

FIGURE 9.3. University of Illinois colonization.

nent centers may be useful to those struggling for perspective. It is offered with hesitation, since interpretations of complex activities are often colored by personal involvement. Jurg Steiger, a physician staff member from the Institute of Research in Medical Education and Evaluation at the University of Bern (Switzerland) Faculty of Medicine, attempted a similar synthesis following a year-long visit to the three centers in 1971-72.[1] His observations and conclusions were not fully endorsed by any of the unit directors; it seems unlikely that I will be able to do any better.

At the time of Steiger's study, each of the three programs had a distinctive flavor, one that had been fashioned by the founding director. By 1978, only at the University of Southern California was that leadership unchanged. At Michigan State, Hilliard Jason resigned as director of OMERAD in 1972. He moved first to the National Library of Medicine for two years as a consultant in medical education, then to the Association of American Medical Colleges as director of a new division. Jason was followed at OMERAD by Ronald Richards who, after a short tenure, moved on to direct a new experimental program of medical education offered by MSU in the upper peninsula of Michigan. Richards was succeeded by Arthur Elstein, whose doctorate is in clinical psychology. A search for his successor was initiated in the later summer of 1979.

At Illinois there was not only a change in directors but also a change in organizational placement. The original Office of Research in Medical Education had already, in 1964, added an outreach arm, which was called the Center for the Study of Medical Education (CSME). As time passed, there was a growing conviction that local educational development could be strengthened and broadened if the Medical Center's campus-wide technical services (instructional television, photography, other audiovisual entities) were merged with the College of Medicine-based ORME/CSME, which would simultaneously broaden its support mission to include the other health professions schools and colleges. Issues of academic territory, authority, and responsibility prevented a total union, but in 1970 a consolidated campus-wide technical service, now called the Office of Educational Resources (OER), and a broadened College of Medicine educational research and development resource, now called the Center for Educational Development (CED), were both placed under my direction. Accountability for OER operation was to the Medical Center chancellor, and for CED functions to the

College of Medicine executive dean. Although authority flowed from two sources, the channeling through a single director made it possible for the two units to be operated as one.

Following a 1972-73 sabbatical leave, I suggested that organizational vigor and effectiveness might be enhanced by new CED/OER leadership. Not until 1974 was that suggestion accepted. The search for a successor was undertaken in 1975, and Philip Forman, a pediatric neurologist turned medical educator, took up the directorship on March 1, 1976.* On the same day William J. Grove, who had been dean and then executive dean of the College of Medicine for eight years, became the first Medical Center vice chancellor for academic affairs. With this reorganization of campus administration, and a new CED/OER director, the time seemed right to complete the long-contemplated shift of axis. In September 1976 a fully consolidated professional/technical resource, now called simply the Center for Educational Development, was established as a campuswide agency under the office of the new vice chancellor.

Today, as in 1971 when Steiger studied them, CED, DRME, and OMERAD are all engaged in educational research, educational service, and training of health professions educators. But the tilt of the tripod, as Steiger saw it, was toward research at Michigan State, toward service (to local faculty) at Southern California, and toward training at Illinois. Such a characterization might not be as evident today as it was at that earlier time, but in one respect it is unchanged: the academic research orientation is probably still more prominent at Michigan State than at either of the others.

This fact, if fact it is, may reflect the early and continuing involvement of distinguished members of Michigan State's College of Education faculty in the work of OMERAD. In neither of the other centers is there anything comparable to the active contributions of a Lee Shulman or a Norman Kagan. Dean Andrew Hunt encouraged this integration of interests and activities; Hilliard Jason, whose joint doctorates in medicine and education facilitated identification with both groups, made it happen; and Arthur Elstein, who absorbed it in his own training, projects an unconcealed personal bent toward fundamental research questions. It is true that Abrahamson also holds a joint appointment in medicine and education, but the inter-

*On December 14, 1978, Dr. Forman was appointed Dean of the Abraham Lincoln School of Medicine in the University of Illinois College of Medicine. The third CED director is Ronald Richards, who had been the second leader of OMERAD at Michigan State.

college collaborative efforts at Southern California have been more evident in training programs than in fundamental research projects. At Illinois the best intentions of collaboration were thwarted by the 130 miles that initially separated the College of Medicine and the College of Education. By the time that distance was shortened to eight city blocks when a second College of Education was established on the Chicago Circle Campus of the University, the patterns of interprofessional communication and support within the Center for Educational Development had been so well established that close and continuing interaction with colleagues in the College of Education never developed.

This is not to suggest that research at Southern California or at Illinois is either less in quantity or inferior in quality to that undertaken at Michigan State; it is simply a reminder that in the first two research is more likely to be applied than basic in nature. Both kinds of systematic study are important, and each contributes to the educational enterprise. While the one approach may win more plaudits in academic circles, the other is usually more treasured by those with urgent problems that demand immediate attention.

In the face of this subtle difference in orientation, it is interesting to note Steiger's conclusion that OMERAD had produced more direct impact on local faculty than either DRME or CED. Such an observation is probably predictable and simply confirms the general feeling that it is easier to fashion a new educational program than to modify an old one. And OMERAD had the unusual opportunity to do this twice: in 1966 when the College of Human Medicine was founded, and again in 1970 when a College of Osteopathic Medicine was established at Michigan State and the educational research and development staff became a part of that program as well.

Recognizing this reality, the Southern California group has generally taken a responsive posture. As Abrahamson put it, "DRME is not involved in decision making or policy making activity . . . our school of medicine faculty includes three basic types: friendlies, neutrals and hostiles. We work closely with the friendlies; we try to influence the neutrals to be more thoughtful about teaching and learning; we are cordial to the hostiles (and hope we are never afflicted with an illness in one of their special areas of interest!)." Over the years this stance has resulted in an untold number of small, and some not so small, changes in the organization or implementation of instructional programs, but nothing at the institutional level as profoundly different as the upper peninsula program at Michigan State.

At Illinois, the Office of Research in Medical Education and its successors were intimately involved in the policy-making apparatus of the College of Medicine, but not with decision making. ORME membership in virtually all the major committees and councils was ex officio, without vote. This absence of authority was an incomparable advantage, since it meant that any program change had been debated and agreed upon by representative faculty groups, not imposed by administrative edict or professional resource dictate. Whatever gains were to be won by ORME could be achieved only through the power of evidence and persuasion. Admittedly these tools were used without reservation, whether in responding to faculty requests for help or in mobilizing faculty concern for educational issues on which help seemed needed, even if not recognized. On at least one major educational policy matter, that of the student evaluation system (which towers above all other curriculum and instruction questions in determining an institutional climate for learning), this approach finally toppled a traditional, punitive, episodic, departmentally-based, memory-oriented system of examinations and replaced it with a professionally staffed, learning/certifying, comprehensive, college-based, and problem-oriented system of student appraisal. Once this learning quality control procedure was in place, it was possible to move on to curriculum changes that emphasized individualized learning opportunities (including one of the earliest independent study programs in medicine), with the ultimate aim of establishing a competency-based rather than a time-based program of study. It was this collegial system of accountability that gave institutional leaders and external accreditation groups some confidence that any disastrously inadequate product would not go undetected when a proposed plan to double the college enrollment and to utilize unfamiliar community settings for education was implemented.

Despite the apparent success of these leading units in facilitating educational change at three medical schools, and the comparable experience of many others, not everyone is convinced of the wisdom of establishing or maintaining such centers. Victor Neufeld at McMaster University has best articulated the challenge. He points out that as they grow larger and acquire more sophisticated, more specialized staff, these units begin to take on a life of their own, one

that may or may not match the needs for which they were originally
established. At the very least, they run the risk of losing identification with the faculty that spawned them. In Neufeld's view there is a
danger that staff interests will become, or at least will seem to become, more important than faculty needs (or wants). Certainly each
of the major centers described here has had to deal with overt or implicit questions about priorities, about the allocation of time and
resources to questions of immediate concern in contrast to those
with a more remote potential payoff, about the appearance that external opportunities have displaced internal responsibilities. Rational arguments on the importance of basic versus applied studies, rea-
reasoned justification for grasping an outside project in order to
strengthen an internal source, and sturdy defense of the essential
need for in-depth training of a few educational professionals over
the superficial exposure of many interested semiprofessionals are
not often persuasive to those who thought they were buying help in
solving their own educational problems, not investing in work that
might improve medical education at large. In some ways this dialogue resembles the contemporary exchange between consumers of
health services and providers. Neufeld suggests that the issue is more
likely to be resolved by improving the educational qualifications of
health professions faculty members themselves, so they can use new
expertise in all their work, than by creating independent professional resource centers to which faculty can turn in the face of need (but
from which they may never get the response they want).

And he may be right. Certainly it was Steiger's view in 1971 that
the most impressive integration of educational science into the work
of a medical school was to be found not in any of those with large
educational centers but at McMaster, which had no formal medical
education research and development unit. It still has only a "Program for Educational Development," which is a coordinated, non-
bureaucratic, functional group drawing collaborators from many
departments to help one another, with the support of research associates rather than leadership by a professional staff.

The issue Neufeld raises does not challenge the desirability of educational research and development in medicine (or, more broadly,
in the health professions); rather it questions the organization and
staffing patterns that will ensure optimal incorporation of that work
into the fabric of a school. Others have raised the question in a dif-

ferent way, one that asks about the role, the responsibilities, and the rewards of those who have made, or are contemplating, a personal investment in this increasingly accepted function that has not yet crystallized into a generally recognized discipline.

At least four groups seem to speak for the function, or at least to represent it, but the sounds that come from them are not identical despite a considerable overlap in their constituency. Probably best known is the assembly of health professionals, basic medical scientists, sociologists, clinical and experimental and educationl psychologists, evaluation specialists, health systems analysts, and others who gather at the annual meeting of the Association of American Medical Colleges under the banner of the Conference on Research in Medical Education. It was here that those interested in the systematic study of medical education first had an opportunity to meet together; to share data, experiences, and frustrations; to gain support from one another; to achieve a sense of identity as well as worth. Seventeen years later the meeting may still serve the same purpose, but it has grown so large that participants must carefully map an optimal path through multiple simultaneous sessions, and make appointments to talk with colleagues who might otherwise never be encountered in the ebb and flow of conference traffic. For the 1978 meeting, 240 contributors were listed in the 475-page multilithed *Proceedings*. That is no small gathering.

The growing size of the Conference on Research in Medical Education, the heterogeneity of the participants, and the variability of their qualifications for discussing issues of concern to leaders in this then new movement contributed to the formation of a second group. It was never formally organized, and members have taken some pride in describing themselves as a "non-group." They are, with few exceptions, directors of medical education units, and their discussions have more often dealt with organizational and administrative matters than with substantive research and development questions. Recurrent themes in these informal exchanges have included the proper organization and placement of such units in the medical school hierarchy, the means of gaining greater recognition for their function (or, in more exuberant moments, their "discipline"), and possible solutions for seemingly endless funding problems. A group such as this might have been expected to mature into a powerful and articulate interpreter of, if not a lobby for, educational research and development in medicine, one that illuminated discrepancies between well-established educational principle and comfortably familiar instructional practice, that identified promising alternatives in educational strategies or tactics, that called attention to new educational opportunities, that generated authoritative commentary on new educational policy proposals. But this small circle never adopted such a role, remaining instead an informal and loosely organized club-like cluster.

Making up a third group were those whose attention was riveted on instructional technology. They had never felt that the Conference on Research in Medical Education really addressed their interests, and their leaders had been consciously excluded from the "nongroup." The most vigorous among them had banded together in a Council on Medical Television, whose regular programs anticipated by half a dozen years the annual AAMC research conference. As other audiovisual technologies became more prominent, the organizational interest also broadened; ultimately it came to embrace a whole spectrum of the types now called biomedical communication specialists in an umbrella group known as the Health Sciences Communication Association. Although their interest is broader than the education of health workers alone, most members are important contributors to that educational enterprise and are not inclined to accept the allegation that their dedication is more to the tools of instruction than to the process of learning. Nevertheless their meetings, certainly more than those of the other groups, do give a good deal of time, space, and attention to the most recent technical refinements of an incredible array of instructional devices, and less attention to research on the educational efficienciey or effectiveness of the equipment that is so dazzling.

Yet none of these coalitions seem to provide a completely comfortable identity for the professionals who have moved from the world of general educational research and development into that of the health professions. The apogee of their world is the American Educational Research Association (AERA). This organization initially had no special place for those who had taken up the new challenge in medicine, but in its constitution there was a provision for the formation of affiliated special interest groups. William Crawford, then a CED staff member, took the initiative to form one. After consulting with colleagues in comparable units, Crawford sounded the call for an organizational meeting in March 1971. By July there were 119 members, and a newsletter had been started. As interest mounted, subsequent annual meetings of this group grew steadily in size and content. By 1976 the Special Interest Group/ Health Professions Education, with 379 members, was the largest within AERA. On the basis of this strength, a move was started to seek recognition as a formal AERA division. This step was taken primarily to gain more program time and greater visibility despite the acknowledged disadvantage of changing "from an informal group with common interests whose primary purpose is facilitating communication, to a structured group which could become embroiled in AERA politics. Our strength lies with the balance between educator-type researchers and clinician-type educators. We would tip the balance toward the educator-type and probably lose the clinician-type. The change may be subtle but it certainly will have a profound effect on how we perceive ourselves."[2]

As it turned out the educator/researcher orientation was preferable to a majority of the membership, and their petition for divisional status was submitted to the AERA Council in 1977. The favorable Council action, taken in 1978, did not produce a Division of Health Professions Education but rather a Division of Education in the Professions, one that could incorporate other groups (such as law, engineering, and theology) with comparable interests. Thus status was gained, but the unique health professions identity was lost, or at the very least substantially diluted.

Four groups, four overlapping but not completely congruent agendas. It would be wrong to challenge the potential contribution of any one of them to the broad mission of educational research and development. The question that only time can answer is whether such alliances will serve the health professions schools and their educational mission, or merely the interests and needs of the members who happen to live and work in those schools.

Although medical schools, or health science centers, have been the primary locus for research and development in health professions education, they are by no means the only sites for such work. During the 1970s comparable efforts were initiated or expanded in many professional organizations.

The *National Board of Medical Examiners* (NBME) is one of the most prominent examples. The worldwide respect now accorded NBME is a tribute to the leadership exercised by John Hubbard for more than a quarter century. Although not himself trained in educational evaluation, Hubbard became the acknowledged spokesman for the application of this emerging discipline to medical education. He was also an enterprising proponent of research and development that broadened both the conceptual framework and the practical utilization of new assessment techniques in the health professions. In the 1950s this work dealt primarily with psychometric refinement of multiple choice examinations, to ensure the highest possible levels of statistical validity and reliability. As the 1960s began, NBME launched a comprehensive research and development program aimed at improving the assessment of clinical competence on completion of an internship. A critical incident study paved the way for definition of that competence; it was followed by the introduction of innovative appraisal techniques (including the first widespread use of programmed examinations, now more commonly referred to as patient management problems). In the early 1970s, the Board established a Committee on Goals and Priorities, whose penetrating analysis and sweeping recommendations[3] set off a series of shock waves that are still rocking the community of medical educators. It is worth noting that the committee was chaired by William Mayer (whose earlier contributions to continuing education and teacher training as a senior administrator in the Division of Regional Medical Programs have already been noted) and included Stephen Abrahamson among its members. This group reaffirmed the importance of an earlier policy statement that identified research in evaluation as an important general program goal, and called for early establishment of a focused and vigorous research division within NBME. The Department of Research and Development, now firmly established and active, is headed by Barbara Andrew (a former University of Southern California DRME staff member); the department's national advisory committee is chaired by Abrahamson, her former chief.

The increasing intensity of NBME research and development is dramatically illustrated in fiscal terms: during the period from 1961 to 1965 the Board received approximately $100,000 in extramural research funds; the figure for 1966 to 1970 was $500,000; and for 1971 to 1976, $1,400,000. In 1977, staff members were engaged in eleven major projects, ranging from investigation of medical record audit and interaction analysis procedures for assessment of physician performance, through computer and audiovisual simulations for assessment of complex cognitive and communication skills, to new adaptations of paper and pencil tests.

Although NBME welcomes the visitors who come from all parts of the world to learn firsthand something more about its work, the unique experience accumulated over more than half a century and the growing and highly qualified professional staff have never been exploited in any organized educational program. The possibility of such a development has been considered by the Board from time to time, and a loose affiliation with CED training activities was even discussed briefly on one occasion. But other demands were more pressing, and no action occurred. In 1976, however, the idea was resurrected by both the policy advisory committee and participants in the annual NBME conference, and the possibility of short-term and collaborative offerings in the principles and practice of health professions educational evaluation is now being actively pursued. March 1979 was set as a target date for completion of a preliminary plan and a proposal for long-term support.

The early contributions made by the *Association of American Medical Colleges* (AAMC) to educational research and development in medicine have already been described, but the further evolution of these endeavors is also a significant part of this story.

The Division of Education, established in 1962 under a Carnegie Foundation grant and Paul Sanazaro's leadership, was organized as a focal point from which the AAMC could encourage the application of educational research findings to ongoing medical education programs; through which consultative services in educational planning and program implementation could be provided to medical schools and professional organizations; and in which basic educational research could be continued and special projects undertaken. These activities were allocated to four functional units. The first area, Educational Research and Services, to which all staff members contributed, included the accumulation and dissemination of descriptive and comparative information about medical schools, the organization and implementation of intramural seminars on medical education, and staff support for the annual conference on research in medical education; the second component, the Office of Basic Research, headed by Edwin Hutchins, continued a long-standing investigation and refinement of the Medical College Admissions Test (MCAT) and a longitudinal study of the class of 1960 in twenty-six medical schools (initiated in 1956 by Helen Hofer

Gee); the third unit, the Office of Student Studies and Services, under Davis Johnson, continued to provide staff support to the Group on Student Affairs (a network that included representatives from each member school) and initiated a definitive study of attrition among American medical students. But it was the fourth area, which Sanazaro chose to call the Core Program, that represented the glimpse of a new future. Regrettably, it did not survive the dissolution of the Division of Education in 1967 and Sanazaro's departure in 1968 to head the USPHS National Center for Health Services Research and Development.

The Core Program included four elements. The first was directed toward delineation of future needs for physicians, as those needs might be influenced by changing demands and functional responsibilities. The second was an effort to establish criteria for acceptable performance of practitioners, to develop suitable measures of performance, to assess performance in selected study samples, and to relate that performance to the educational programs through which the practitioners had passed. The third component was designed to define and document the nature of teaching programs in comprehensive medicine, a topic that only then was beginning to achieve the popularity it has now won. The final element was simply called research in patient care; it was both described and justified in a *Journal of Medical Education* editorial that said in part:

> The ultimate purpose of clinical teaching programs is to teach students and physicians what they must know and do if they are to provide patient care in the best modern meaning of the term. The effectiveness of these programs is judged by the extent to which they attain this objective. The objective in turn must be stated in explicit criteria of the adequacy and appropriateness of patient care. The analogy between "teaching students" and "caring for patients" may clarify the cardinal principle of validation against external criteria.
>
> Learning by students is often equated with the teaching to which they are exposed. Similarly patient care is commonly equated with diagnosis and treatment. But teaching is not identical with learning, nor is diagnosing and treating identical with patient care. The effectiveness of teaching is determined by the objectively measured learning of the student, and the effectiveness of clinical skills (diagnosing and treating) can only be determined by objectively measured responses of the patient.

It is commonplace to measure learning according to the objectively specifiable categories of knowledge and understanding, skills (psychomotor and intellectual), and attitudes and interests. Medical educators utilize this conceptual system daily in assessing student performance. But the evidence available in the studies of Osler Peterson, Kenneth Clute, and Phillip Price and associates, suggests that there is presently no necessary correlation between grades of students in medical school and their later professional performance as practitioners. That is, current teaching of patient care has so far not been validated against actual measures of patient care. Perhaps this tells us that there needs to be some modification in what we as faculty members believe is important for the student to know and to do for the welfare of his future patient.[4]

The editorial went on to call for accelerated research in patient care, research that would lead to the establishment of criteria for determining the adequacy of that care, since such criteria are "essential for the rational design of contemporary curricula in clinical medicine." As an AAMC contribution to this effort, the Division of Education launched a series of seminars on the subject. These seminars took as a model "prior experience with the seminars on medical teaching (that) enabled a significant number of faculty members to channel their interest in teaching more effectively by assisting them to identify the major principles which should guide them in designing and evaluating their own teaching efforts."

With Sanazaro's departure from the AAMC, this visionary effort to link the medical education system with the medical care system withered on an untended vine. The educational consultation service suffered a similar fate. In 1971-72 a Division of Curriculum and Instruction emerged to fill the gap, but this program was shortly replaced by a Division of Educational Resources. The new program was devoted primarily to a joint project with the National Library of Medicine aimed at fostering the more effective use of instructional hardware, and a more systematic and objective evaluation of instructional software. A successful undertaking, the project led, among other things, to the establishment of a now widely used computer-based system called AVLine for retrieval of information about audiovisual software.

During these years, members of the "non-group" of medical education unit leaders were mounting a campaign for more integral involvement in the work of the AAMC. The Division of Educational Measurement, one of the successors to the earlier Office of Basic Research and the division now responsible for the annual conference on research on medical education, responded in 1971 by initiating the formation of a nationally representative assembly of medical school personnel involved with research on, and implementation/evaluation of, the process of medical education. The model for this new organizational alliance was the standing Group on Student Affairs composed of student affairs officers from each member school. As it turned out, the Group on Medical Education (GME) that emerged from this effort had among its members neither the homogeneity of professional backgrounds and responsibilities nor the identity of interests that characterized the Group on Student Affairs. Those nominated by individual school deans were apparently selected on the basis of general interest in educational problems, administrative responsibility for some portion of the academic program, or faculty responsibility for chairing a key educational committee, but relatively few of them proved to be professionally trained or experientially qualified in educational research and development. Although the GME has provided a useful forum for discussion of educational questions at both national and regional levels, it has rarely measured up to the educational research and development promise envisioned by those who had pressed most vigorously for its establishment.

These early shakers and movers also made known their belief that the *Journal of Medical Education* should reflect the orientation of those directly involved in educational research and development as well as that of the program administrators (the deaning types) and academic scholars (the biomedical research types) who then dominated the editorial board. John Cooper, *Journal* editor and AAMC president, responded (in a manner reminiscent of the Teaching Institute evolution) by appointing in 1971 a distinguished medical sociologist, Renee Fox, as the first representative of this new breed. She was followed one year later by Ralph Ingersoll and Hilliard Jason, both directors of medical school education units. Today, four of the nineteen editorial board members are primarily identified with medical education research and development programs.

The boldest move, following the disappearance of the Division of Education, was taken in 1974 when a Division of Faculty Development was established and Hilliard Jason was appointed to head it.

The Division's goals were: (1) to identify areas of difficulty or deficiency in the design and implementation of medical education programs, with particular attention paid to the effectiveness of faculty members; (2) to devise strategies for providing assistance in the correction of deficiencies and the solution of educational problems; (3) to identify, mobilize, and cultivate resources for assisting faculty members to enlarge their understanding of educational issues, and to enhance their competence in educational design and implementation.

Although the words were different, the music was not unlike that which had launched the Division of Education more than ten years earlier. As with that prior program, a vigorous plan for action accompanied the delineation of these admirable goals. The plan included establishment of short-term faculty workshops on various educational topics, creation of long-term training opportunities for faculty leaders, development of instructional packages, dissemination of information and ideas drawn from educational research and demonstration projects, liaison with university-based faculty development programs, and provision of educational consultation services to medical schools. Before these varied activities could be fully launched, however, Division staff members were caught up in work aimed at fulfillment of the first program goal: identification of areas of educational deficiency or difficulty.

The Faculty Development Survey, which occupied so much staff time, was a remarkable study. It elicited from a stratified random sample of 2,700 medical school faculty members in the United States (drawn from a total population of 27,393) information on their preparation for teaching (through forced choice questions), their instructional practices in dealing with common educational problems (as presented in written simulations), and the kind of external assistance they would be willing to accept in finding better solutions to these problems (through forced choice questions). The findings were both discouraging and encouraging, depending on whether the point of reference was the ideal toward which we had been aiming for twenty years, or the point from which things had begun.[5] For example, in 1977 "only 21% have taken courses in education and only 39% have ever attended an educational workshop." A long way to go, but a mighty step beyond what things were like in 1957. Even more encouraging was the evidence that large numbers of faculty respondents were, if not eager, at least ready to accept help in improving their instructional skills. Although most expressed a strong preference for turning to colleagues for this help, many more than would have accepted the suggestion twenty years earlier were now ready to use specialists in educational process or printed materials as aids to self-improvement.

On the basis of these findings and the experience gained in a series of pilot workshops that involved some 358 faculty members from 94 medical schools, the Division of Faculty Development planned to move ahead with the creation of instructional self-assessment packages for medical teachers and workshops on the process and content of faculty development for those who carried this responsibility in member schools (in contrast to the originally proposed educational topic workshops for faculty members themselves). But before these important thrusts could be implemented, a decision to phase out this newest AAMC division was made. It sounded very much like history repeating itself, but this time the program was to continue in another setting. The announcement of change stated simply that the Association and the program sponsors (the Kellogg Foundation and the Commonwealth Fund) were agreed that a university would provide a better laboratory for this work and thus would be a more suitable base of operation. On July 1, 1978, the new National Center for Faculty Development, under Jason's direction, opened at the University of Miami School of Medicine. Its function and its future remain to be seen.

Most readers will know that such activities as those described here represent only a small part of AAMC work. Certainly in recent years major attention has been given, for example, to a very successful management development program for medical school administrators; to a smoothly functioning and influential interaction with the federal agencies that now have such profound impact on medical centers; to a continuing effort to broaden and strengthen support for biomedical research; to facilitation of communication among the several constituencies of academic health science centers. All of these accomplishments deserve high praise. However, they cannot conceal the undeniable ambivalence that has marked AAMC interest in the educational process itself over the last fifteen years. The termination of two major undertakings that addressed not merely the structure of educational programs or the tools of instruction, but also the purposes of that education and the performance of educators, is only one example, although perhaps the most dramatic, of uncertainty about organizational role and responsibility in this field. The provision of a forum for exchange of research nd development reports has been a commendable achievement, but in drawing back from direct involvement in research and development activities that might demand new action, changed values, and altered faculty behavior, the AAMC may have to be faulted.

The *American Medical Association* (AMA) has eased into the turbulent waters of educational research and development on only a few occasions, but they were important events even if short-lived.

The first venture was stimulated by Ward Darley's 1961 call for the establishment of a National Academy of Continuing Education, a university without walls that would mount a comprehensive program to narrow the widening gap between an accelerating growth of medical knowledge and its incorporation into the daily work of medical practitioners.[6] With notable vision and commendable leadership, the American Medical Association took up the gauntlet flung down by the Association of American Medical Colleges and mobilized six other professional groups to join with the AMA and AAMC as sponsors of an effort to generate a workable plan. The resulting Joint Study Committee (consisting of John Z. Bowers, chairman; R. H. Kampmeier, John P. Lindsay, George E. Miller, and Samuel P. Newman; with C. H. William Ruhe [AMA] and J. Frank Whiting [AAMC] as staff members) selected Bernard Dryer as study director. His final report, "Lifetime Learning for Physicians,"[7] a conceptual and practical blueprint for action, was presented to the sponsors in March 1962. The report was accepted and the study committee was encouraged to move toward implementation of the concepts set forth there. Unfortunately, that encouragement was not accompanied by the funds required for action.

Nevertheless, the idea for a "National Plan" was kept alive in the AMA Department of Postgraduate Programs. There, under the leadership of Patrick Storey, general strategy and specific tactics began to take shape. It was not, however, the shape of a highly sophisticated communications network which many had seen as the ultimate thrust of Dryer's recommendations (although Dryer himself had specifically warned against the oversimplified view that continuing education was merely a matter of getting the latest information to the doctor by the fastest route possible). Instead, Storey, with his colleagues John Williamson and Hilman Castle, brought the focus back to the basic objective of continuing medical education:

to improve the quality of medical care delivered by practitioners. Their plan recognized the central importance of integrating continuing education with daily practice (in contrast to the usual classroom spirit of conventional programs), of beginning with specification of educational objectives (derived from identified deficiencies in medical care), of designing learning experiences aimed specifically at correcting these deficiencies, and of incorporating an evaluation procedure to determine whether the effort to improve medical care had been achieved through the instructional effort. It was, in fact, a highly pragmatic application of the principles of learning and program organization long espoused by educational scientists.

Between 1963 and 1966, the conceptual plan was refined, the study instruments developed, the instructional methods elaborated, and pilot programs carried out. The report of that work was an exciting chapter in the history of continuing medical education,[8] but the world of medicine was apparently not ready for a national plan that required diagnosis of educational need before administration of educational therapy. As it turned out, physicians approached continuing education in much the same way that so many patients approached health care: they preferred a familiar remedy that promised to do no harm and might do some good rather than submitting first to an uncomfortable, sometimes threatening, diagnostic workup. Despite premature termination, this effort was in important step in the long path toward transforming programs of continuing medical education into something that exploited, rather than neglected, sound principles of learning.

Although this national plan was never fully implemented, William Ruhe, then director of the Division of Education and now senior vice president of the AMA, recognized the importance of introducing a larger number of health professionals trained in education, as well as in medicine, into the system of continuing education program planning, implementation, and evaluation. As a result of his intervention, from 1969 to 1974 the AMA provided fellowships in medical education for one or two trainees each year at the University of Illinois Center for Educational Development. That support was brought to an end not by conceptual disillusionment but by the fiscal constraints that affected many AMA activities during the mid-1970s.

Two of these fellows were part of an additional AMA educational research and development program. The project grew naturally out of the ill-fated national plan and reflected the continuing interest in the principles on which it had been based. If diagnosis of need was to precede prescription of educational therapy, further perfection of diagnostic tools was an essential element in the process. To address this problem a collaborative Physician Self-Assessment Study was undertaken from 1972 to 1974. The original grant application outlined a three-year cooperative endeavor between the AMA and CED to develop and test several alternatives. The two-year study that was finally funded focused on designing and testing printed and computerized simulations of clinical encounters alone. The work proved to be an impressive exploitation of available technology, one that succeeded in exciting a significant number of physicians who contributed to the instructional content and in so doing became familiar with the educational process. The pilot studies also provided interesting information about the ways in which generalists and specialists, older and more recent graduates, attacked and resolved the sample problems — and at what cost. Although it was not possible to continue this developmental project beyond termination of external support, the AMA Division of Education has maintained an interest in documenting and encouraging further work on this vital element of sound individualized continuing education.

It is in this area of testing that other professional organizations have been most active in educational research and development, often in collaboration with organizations such as the National Board of Medical Examiners or with other educational consultants. Initially the self-assessment test procedures that came out of these efforts were little more than multiple-choice probes of current information recall; today many deal with higher level cognitive performance, and some have even attempted to assess psychomotor skills. At last count (September 1978), thirty specialty societies had followed the lead of the American College of Physicians in offering self-assessment programs to members and often to others as well. It is unfortunate that so few have capitalized on this opportunity to study the professional performance strengths and weaknesses of physicians, to determine how (or whether) continuing education programs alter performance patterns, and to report these findings in the medical education literature.

Medical specialty boards, or their related professional societies, have also picked up the practice of offering diagnostic examinations as an aid to individual resident learning and assessment of residency programs. Since they were first used by the American Board of Orthopaedic Surgery in 1963, annual or biennial in-training examinations have been developed by ten other specialty groups. But as with the physician self-assessment tests, the results have been used almost entirely for personal and private feedback to trainees and program directors. Although such knowledge is useful to those receiving the information, it contributes nothing to the solution of important questions about individual rates of learning, the influence of instructional methods and training sites on achievement, or the concurrent and predictive validity of the tests themselves, among other things. It is another example of incorporating sound educational principles but losing the research and development opportunity such action provides.

It would be unfortunate to stop here, leaving the impression from these illustrations that assimilation and integration have occurred only in the United States, for that is far from true. As a matter of fact, the science of education has probably been incorporated more fully in at least a few new basic professional programs in other countries than in almost any U.S. medical school founded during the last ten years. Among the notable examples are the Ben Gurion University of the Negev in Israel; the McMaster Faculty of Medicine in Canada; the Maastricht Faculty of Medicine in the Netherlands; the Xochimilcho Faculty of the Autonomous Metropolitan University of Mexico City; and most recently, the University of Newcastle in Australia. All of these schools, and others like them, have gone at least one step beyond the applications of educational science that were stressed during the early years of this work. It is a step that has rarely been taken in the United States.

This further direction was implicit in Paul Sanazaro's core program and was spelled out with great elegance in his presentation to the 1966 AMA Congress on Medical Education.[9] It has probably been articulated most forcefully in recent times by Tamas Fulop, director of the WHO Division of Health Manpower Development, in the course of analyzing the achievements and limitations of the global health professions teacher training program, whose success few would deny. Essentially his questions run this way: Has educational science, as it is now applied, changed the fundamental nature of medical education or merely helped teachers and learners to achieve more efficiently and effectively goals that are of secondary rather than of primary importance? Is anything of real significance gained if teachers specify more precisely, and in behavioral terms, learning objectives that have only a remote relationship to the real world of health care? Is anything important achieved if new curriculum organization or instructional methodology merely help students to learn more rapidly about problems they will rarely encounter as practitioners? Is it really helpful for faculties to evaluate with ever greater statistical validity and reliability student knowledge and skills that are of no more than peripheral importance in the health care most needed by the populations they must serve?

Although such questions were generated by concern for a growing gap between the things medical school graduates are prepared to do and the health care problems of developing nations, they have the strange ring of truth for developed nations as well. The rebellious student demands for relevance in education voiced in the 1960s are now being echoed by thoughtful health professions faculty leaders, who find conventional academic values increasingly out of touch with reality in the contemporary world. But relevance now refers not so much to the immediate utility of what is taught or learned day by day or week by week, as to the congruence between educational programs, community needs, and available resources. The present mismatch has been captured with exquisite sensitivity and feeling in the opening chapter of John Bryant's book *Health and the Developing World*. With less passion, but equal conviction, his preface establishes the tone of what follows, saying:

> Large numbers of the world's people, perhaps more than half, have no access to health care at all, and for many of the rest the care they receive does not answer the problems they have. The grim irony is that dazzling advances in biomedical science are scarcely felt in areas where the need is greatest . . . Whatever the desires of nations to reach their people with health care, the actual task of doing so is extraordinarily difficult. It is difficult in Malawi, one of the world's poorest countries, so is it difficult in the United States, one of the world's richest . . .
>
> In most countries, unfortunately, health care is seriously inadequate, which reflects not only on poverty of resources but also on both the design of the system and the education of the health personnel. Indeed, in going from country to country and looking, on the one hand, at the large and complex health care programs and related educational institutions and, on the other hand, at the pitifully limited benefits reaching the

majority of people, the unavoidable impression emerges of great but unavailing effort.[10]

In the World Health Organization, at least, such views have not diminished concern for improving the pedagogic qualifications of health professions faculty members, but they have spurred efforts to consolidate that work with attempts to improve the health service delivery system. This is being done by bringing the educators of health personnel and the providers of health services together, to work cooperatively and in tandem toward a common goal of improving health (and medical) care. Implicit before, that goal is being made explicit in a unitary Health Services and Manpower Development program.

So it has come to pass that a new set of words and phrases has begun to enter the vocabulary of educational planners wherever they gather. There is less talk about integration and correlation of individual disciplines and more about problem-based and competency-based and community-oriented curriculum organization, about mastery learning and interdisciplinary and interprofessional study, for example. The focus is shifting from preoccupation with academic content and instructional methods to professional performance goals and health care outcomes. Both the academic specialist and the professional educator are beginning to sense that a major change is once more near.

PROBLEMS AND PROSPECTS

10

When directors of educational research and development programs were invited, in the 1977 questionnaire, to identify any significant impediments to the work of their units, the responses were varied, usually thoughtful, and often suggested frustration stemming from a perceived inability to reduce or circumvent the obstacles they cited. One new incumbent replied with a hint of irony, "If I tried to take an objective look at impediments to getting my program off the ground, I would probably quit." From most respondents, however, the major areas of concern fell into one of three broad categories: funding, recognition, and rewards.

Very few medical school departments ever feel that the funds available for their support match the importance of their work or the extent of their responsibilities. The resulting interdepartmental conflict over money, though never stilled, is generally tolerable during periods of institutional growth; but in a no-growth phase, or in a time of declining institutional support, this conflict may reach the level of internecine warfare. Today many medical schools find themselves in just such a situation—their research dollars dwindling, the training grants shrinking, federal capitation awards reduced, and, in the face of a brewing taxpayer revolt, appropriations made with increasing caution by state legislators. And all this at a time when the cost of everything is rising.

Medical education units certainly share this fiscal problem with other medical school departments, but because they are often among the most recent additions to the institutional community, the pinch may be particularly acute. Many such programs have not yet been fully integrated into the regular internal budget schema, and the external sources of educational research and development grants and contracts, which were never plentiful, have diminished even more rapidly than those in biomedical science. Among the thirty-three questionnaire respondents who provided the fiscal information requested, certainly those five who reported that more than 70 percent of their support came from federal capitation funds, and the twelve who noted that more than 50 percent of the operating budget was derived from soft money sources, may face serious trouble. The larger units can probably survive a sharp reduction in funding, though at the expense of program diversity and depth, but for smaller units any significant erosion of support may lead to such a contraction of core staff that effective function will be compromised.

In the intramural battle for budget, education units may also be disadvantaged because of a second problem, one that has been labeled recognition. The point is sometimes made by explicit faculty complaints that these units are siphoning off funds that might better be used for the more important work of advancing the biomedical sciences. More often, however, the lack of recognition is simply manifested as apathy toward, or outright hostility to, a discipline that is poorly understood and generally looked upon as soft, if not actually mushy. One acute observer put it this way:

> The new discipline moved into the medical milieu as did Cortez on the Indians. The educationists sometimes seemed to possess intuitively a great truth far above the ineptness of the jugglers of hours and schedules. They used a language which though new and appealing was in essence meaningless to the uninitiated. Such phrases as "the learning environment," "information versus knowledge," "data base versus facts," "behavioral endpoints," "educational objectives" were often abrasive rather than soothing. The lack of communication created by the jargon polarized the opinions of the Indians. A few were attracted; a few were hostile; but most were unimpressed, skeptical, or indifferent.[1]

If lack of recognition by faculty members creates a problem for educational units, that problem is magnified manyfold when the indifference or skepticism is shared by the dean. Since the tenure of medical school deans now averages less than three years, even a sympathetic and supportive leader may be gone before the educational research and development program is firmly rooted. Moreover, there is never any guarantee that a successor will exhibit comparable enthusiasm for what is still not universally regarded as central to the institutional mission.

But it is the third problem, the reward system, that was noted most frequently, and with the greatest feeling, as a major impediment to program development. Although salary limitations were mentioned by a few, most of those who identified this obstacle were referring to the less tangible academic rewards that have their most visible manifestation in promotion to higher academic ranks. The inescapable fact appears to be that most medical schools simply do not know how to deal with this new species. A few institutions have solved the problem by giving educational research and development staff members purely administrative or functional titles. However, most schools recognize that professional personnel, contributing directly to academic programs, expect and often demand an academic appointment. Since fewer than one-third of the educational units can themselves award academic rank, some alternative arrangement has been sought. It has usually taken the form of nominal appointment in another sympathetic department—medicine, pediatrics, anatomy, microbiology—which may solve the immediate problem but creates another when promotion time approaches. In practice, even accepting the best of intentions (which do not always exist), it is unrealistic to expect a promotions committee of microbiologists or pediatricians to judge the quality of research carried out in a foreign discipline that uses unfamiliar methods, or to evaluate the general contributions to that discipline made by an educationist. The situation is further complicated by the fact that these professionals often devote much of their time to fulfilling the consultation and service demands made by medical school departments and individual faculty members (in curriculum organization, instructional materials development, or evaluation design and implementation), leaving them little opportunity for research, which is the surest path to academic recognition and promotion.

Some might say this plight is no different from that of a physiologist, who has to spend most of his time teaching, or a pediatrician, who must give most of her time to patient care. To the extent that such a common problem exists, it requires attention and correction. But there is one significant difference in dealing with the educationist who has chosen to work in a medical school: such individuals have other choices. They do not need to leave the familiar academic setting of their own discipline where they can work on problems that match more closely those encountered in their training, and where their contributions can be judged (and rewarded) by peers who understand what they are trying to do. Unquestionably the challenge of medical education has an inherent excitement that appeals to an ever-increasing number of professionals from the world of education, but if educational research and development are to prosper in schools for the health professions, the challenge must be accompanied by appropriate recognition and reward. If not, it will wither or be left to those who cannot make a mark in the conventional educational career they were prepared to enter.

Without minimizing the importance of these impediments identified by educational unit leaders, an alternative interpretation of their observations is also possible. It may be that problems of funding, recognition, and rewards are merely disabling symptoms of more pervasive disorders within the medical education system or among the medical education research and development practitioners. Although such a diagnosis may be uncomfortable, it is at least worth considering.

Turning first to *system problems,* few observers would deny that medical faculties are dominated by basic and clinical scientists whose first loyalty is advancement of the discipline with which they are identified. However, any dispassionate analyst would also acknowledge that a faculty member really has two disciplines—one biomedical, the other educational. Yet the spirit of scientific inquiry, which should characterize both, seems generally to be left in the laboratory when it is time to move to the classroom. Curiously, this discrepancy is rarely recognized, and even less frequently verbalized. Scientists who refuse to accept Krebiozen or Lactrile on the basis of testimonials see nothing strange about embracing methods of instruction and evaluation whose use is supported by nothing more substantial. Investigators who insist that systematic study of biologic phenomena, rather than individual experience, must be the base from which to draw conclusions see nothing inconsistent in any rejection of carefully planned educational studies whose findings fail to match their personal preferences. Medical teachers seem quite prepared to accept data that support the educational views they hold but are strangely unresponsive to findings that suggest a need for change in the way they do things. Arrogance may be too strong a word to describe this behavior, but it is certainly closer to reality than the spirit of inquiry that is always claimed as the hallmark of higher professional education. Humility can surely be learned, but it cannot be taught by teachers who provide the model in only that part of their lives given to the academic pursuit of a biomedical discipline. Unless some diffidence is also integrated into their instructional role, students will get a mixed message about its worth; and, incidentally, educational scientists will have limited opportunity to test in medicine the utility of what they espouse.

A second system problem may lie in the conflict of values that is imposing an ever-increasing strain upon the higher education establishment. Growing out of the British vision of a gentlemanly community of scholars and the German model of a graduate education/research institute, the American university amalgam continues to prize individual scholarly study, which has as its goal the expansion of human knowledge without reference to its social value. The unique contribution to higher education that has come from the New World was introduced little more than a century ago through the land-grant institution, whose mission was to harness the potential of scholarly work for the practical betterment of agriculture and industry. This pragmatic orientation was even captured in the seal of the University of Illinois, which conveys a commitment to "Learning and Labor," a sharp contrast to the seal of Harvard University, which says quite simply "Veritas." But as the years have passed and many of the early land-grant colleges have grown into giant multiversities, the trend has been increasingly toward the search for eternal truth rather than temporal utility, toward research more properly characterized as pure than applied, toward academic work that can be admired for its technical elegance rather than applauded for its practical worth.

In such a climate it is relatively easy for authorities in disparate disciplines to live and work in geographic proximity. The tie that binds them is a common commitment to pursue knowledge, with the implicit understanding that what is found in one college, school, or department will not necessarily affect what is done in another. Thus professors of medicine, surgery, and psychiatry can all study the problem of peptic ulcer, and can in the same university hospital treat the patients chance assigns to them by smoothing the ragged crater with antacids, soothing the frayed psyche with insight, or cutting the evil out. Although they may privately (and sometimes publicly) berate one another for such behavior, there is no expectation that the studies by one group will perforce influence the practices of another.

Research conducted in academic schools of education may be perceived in the same way — as something that is important to educators, but not anything that is expected to influence other disciplines. The educational research and development carried out in medical schools, on the other hand, has action as its goal, not simply the accumulation of knowledge that may at some future time influence decisions. It is intended to make explicit the educational goals and objectives that are usually implicit, to assure a match between these objectives and the curriculum organization/learning climate, to enhance faculty skill in the use of instructional tools and evaluation procedures, to document educational outcomes in terms of specified intent. The purpose is to improve the educational process and product (learning and labor), not simply to illuminate or elucidate what exists (*veritas*). It would be difficult for a faculty to deny that both kinds of research are legitimate, but to paraphrase George Orwell: All research is equal, but some kinds of research are more equal than others.

A third system impediment to the integration of educational research into educational program development is the academic tradition of departmental autonomy, a tradition that is sometimes even more jealously guarded than that of tenure. Departmental status is an overt acknowledgment of disciplinary maturity and independent position. It is as eagerly sought by the protagonists of a new body of knowledge (or the promotion of an old subdivision) as by an adolescent feeling the thrust of new hormones. Once established, a department next demands instructional time which, when gained, is protected against invasion with a ferocity that often transforms academic curriculum committee meetings into battlefields where winners get the largest bundle of hours.

Joseph Wearn and his associates at Western Reserve mounted the first contemporary attack by a medical school on this dominant principle of institutional organization. It was a shining example of the way leaders can establish new linkages and combinations in the interest of basic professional education while preserving the departmental structure for graduate education and research. But even in that setting, recidivism soon set in among clinical departments. Many other schools that made similar efforts were less successful in breaking down old patterns or simply succeeded in setting up new alliances which developed territorial imperatives like those that had characterized the earlier departments.

The problem is not one of territorial battles alone, however; it also involves the quality of life lived within that space. Very few schools have managed to establish any effective system for continuously monitoring anything more than the content of instructional programs; and even here the effort has been sporadic and attended by indifferent success. For the most part, once time has been assigned a department organizes its own course of instruction, one that is believed to be consistent with whatever institutional goals have been established and with the current disciplinary view of what is important to teach. In accordance with the contemporary academic value system, the important things are usually the new things—the cutting edge of a discipline more often than the parts dulled by long use.

It would be hard to fault a department for wanting to familiarize students with recent advances if it were not for two other considerations. The first is that in dwelling upon what is new and challenging to them, teachers may neglect what is old and represents the base upon which understanding of recent developments must rest. Faculty members are inclined to respond to this charge by assuring critics that they do not attempt to teach all the new facts, merely the principles. However, without the checks and balances that external scrutiny provides, it is sometimes difficult to distinguish the one from the other.

A second and more significant consideration is the growing recognition that what most needs to be acquired in medical school is not a vast body of knowledge, much of which will be outmoded by graduation, but a set of attitudes and values that will persist throughout a professional career. There is much talk about the central importance of having students gain a commitment to lifelong learning, a sense of personal responsibility for that learning, a spirit of critical inquiry, a sensitivity to individual human needs, and a willingness to share decision making with patients rather than denying them an opportunity to have a voice in determining how their health shall be maintained or their ill health managed. Yet attitudes of this sort cannot be picked up in a course, nor can they be instilled by one department; they must permeate every part of an institutional program, with continuous reinforcement and reward.

It is here that the medical educationist, charged to assist faculty in designing a curriculum, instructional materials, or evaluation procedures that address such goals, often experiences the greatest frustration. Despite individual concern for the importance of these outcomes, the virtually autonomous departments, preoccupied with content coverage, too often prefer to leave these less tangible matters to someone else. What should be everybody's business becomes nobody's business, in spite of persuasive evidence that such behavior not only fails to support the achievement of these attitudinal goals but may actually defeat their fulfillment.

Turning now to *educational practitioner problems,* it is helpful to begin with the Eighth Annual Conference on Research in Medical Education, held in 1969, which opened on a reflective note, an effort to gain perspective by looking back, looking around, and looking ahead. The keynote address opened with a "reluctant conclusion that the steadily accelerating educational research effort during the last decade has exhibited more promise than direct influence upon educational programs for medical students, interns, residents, and practitioners." After examining the institutional and attitudinal reasons why this might be so, the argument went on in this fashion:

Let me then turn finally to us — the research workers — to who we are and what we do. It must be quickly evident to anyone who examines our backgrounds that we are a motley crew. We come from such diverse disciplines as clinical medicine and basic medical science, experimental psychology and educational psychology, sociology and anthropology, statistics and communications. We share no common training experience and no common goals, other than a general inclination to do good for medical education; we are bound together by no certifying body and have met no special requirements for the practice of our craft: in fact the one thing which we seem to share is an interest in research (which happens to take medical education as its field of focus) far more than a concern for education (which takes research as a means toward action). This may be our glory but I have the uncomfortable feeling that it is our problem. If I may now make some judgments I would be inclined to say that we are too concerned with the trappings of science and not enough with its spirit, that we are more concerned with the legitimacy of our work than with the impact it may have; more concerned with the accumulation of new data than the exploitation of old truth; more concerned with the study of little things that can be controlled than with the exploration of large things that have meaning; more concerned with our individual projects than with the educational systems in which they are carried out. We are in fact very much like the biomedical research workers who grew strong in their science over a twenty year period but are now in the midst of a painful discovery that they have lost touch with their constituency. In no way does this lessen the quality of their work or their personal competence, but it has significantly sapped their support.[2]

The circumstances that led to such a view have undergone little change in the ensuing ten years, but if change has occurred it may be further movement in the same direction rather than any retreat from that position. Many more people are now involved in the medical education research and development enterprise, yet it is difficult to avoid a feeling that the growth in numbers has been accompanied by a growth in professionalism, one that identifies these workers ever more closely with those committed primarily to microcosmic studies (the AERA orientation). If anything, there has been a slow decline in the earlier aggressive efforts to apply old and new knowledge of educational process to the broad problems medicine faces, not merely to the narrow instructional questions of immediate concern to faculty members (or even worse, of interest to professional educators alone). Although this may be the path toward academic legitimacy, it is probably not the way to bring about significant change. As another observer has put it:

> The medical schools are being forced to answer the question: "education for what?" Unfortunately educational research is neither attuned to the pressures nor capable of responding to them and helping medical faculties out of the predicament. The social pressures may be staved off by the methods at hand but they cannot be eliminated by this means. Educational research is using a scalpel where a plow is needed; we are applying sophisticated methodologies to trivial matters, producing results of limited use instead of inquiring into the very fundamental assumptions which form the basis of our current education system.[3]

It is this seeming isolation of the medical education research and development community from the world that medical education is intended to serve, their apparent unfamiliarity with the problems medical practitioners must face, and their ostensible reluctance to voice bold views that may, in the end, prove to be the greatest threat to further integration of this work into the fabric of medicine. The kinds of studies now being done will almost certainly continue, and will continue to be helpful. Some of the weaker institutional units may not survive, but it seems unlikely that any will thrive without re-direction of a significant portion of the total effort, and reaffirmation of the intimate collaboration between educational and health professionals with which the work began.

What, then, of the future?

It is not as though the leaders of medical education units and the individuals who staff them have been without thoughtful advice on questions that their work might most profitably address. That friendly philistine, Edmund Pellegrino, began his review of the situation in 1970 by saying, "The first decade of serious research in medical education appears to have accomplished much of value . . . During the current era researchers have understandably concentrated on what is closest at hand: the immediate experience of students in the medical schools." His "but . . ." was followed by an elegant account of the social changes that had by then placed medical education in a public spotlight where all its warts as well as its beauty lay exposed, subject to analysis and dissection. In this context, Pellegrino concluded that "For the immediate future we must give attention to those questions that bear closely on some of the social and public uses of medicine . . . Effective evaluation research, if it is to produce change, must do so on the basis of observations directed to the suitability of a curricular mode in producing physicians adapted to the major social uses of medicine."[4]

More recently Richard Magraw and his associates, reporting the deliberations of a Work Group on the Education of the Health Professions and the Nation's Health, also noted that "most research on professional education involves examining the effectiveness of the teaching and learning process without questioning whether either makes a significant difference in the health of individuals and groups."[5] As Pellegrino had done earlier, this group then went on to outline a research agenda for the future, one that demands thoughtful consideration by those most directly responsible for medical education research and development programs. The agenda included seven items which suggest that research *should:*

1. Address relationships between what is learned in health professions education and the effect of professional intervention

on the care of individual patients and the health status of the American people.

2. Examine health services and the health status of people in different regions and cultures in relation to variations in health professions education and practice.

3. Address the lack of attention to preventive health measures in health professions education and professional practice and by the public.

4. Address the effect of educational programs aimed at diminishing professional and disciplinary insularity on practice patterns and, subsequently, on the health status of the population served.

5. Identify contributions of education and practice to professional behavior and their effect on health status and relief from discomfort.

6. Relate financing and reimbursement policies for education and practice to the educational system, practice patterns, and health status.

7. Provide a better understanding of how health services research can influence changes in education practices, health status, and relief from discomfort.

One can almost hear gasps of incredulity and cries of "Who, us?" from the educational psychologists, test and measurement specialists, curriculum design personnel, and instructional technology experts, as well as the conventionally trained basic and clinical scientists, who now populate medical education units. It is an understandable question, but it should produce an unequivocally positive response. Present personnel may not be able to accomplish these goals alone, and they will probably need to acquire new knowledge, new skills, and new attitudes before tackling such objectives. But they cannot ignore the need for a redirection of energy and effort. The study of education *qua* education—continuing in a health professions setting the kind of work that might be mounted in a school of education—is no longer enough. New thrusts inevitably strain an established system, but at a time when talk of interprofessional work and matrix organization is so common, it may be useful to remember that educational research and development in medicine has for twenty-five years claimed to be an interdisciplinary collaborative effort built around problems that needed solving, not simply content that needed dissemination. The cast of characters and the nature of those problems may change, but the process can only be strengthened by the infusion of new blood and the struggle with new challenges.

However, research is only one of the objectives a medical education unit is expected to address. In fact, if an average faculty member were asked to list the functional responsibilities of such an organization, educational research would probably rank well below the provision of such technical services as curriculum planning, preparation of instructional modules, production of audiovisual materials, and the construction, scoring, and reporting of examinations. This perception is frequently accompanied by an expectation that the unit will exhibit a responsive posture, much like that of a clinical laboratory, and will perform the services requested without question or comment. For technical staff members this expectation may pose no problem; but for those who regard themselves as academic professionals, it is perceived as demeaning and unworthy. A professional staff is usually willing, often eager, to deliver technical services, but as part of a professional resource function.

A professional resource, like a technical service, may also operate in a responsive mode, but not one that is unquestioning. Faculty should come to such a resource with educational problems to be solved, not with preconceived answers and an expectation that their predetermined remedy will be served up on demand. In dealing with a professional resource, the teacher who asks for help in making an instructional videotape, for example, must expect to be confronted by a series of questions (phrased, one would hope, with tact rather than challenge) that seek to identify the learning objective to be served, the audience to be addressed, the content to be covered, and the alternative strategies that might be employed. Medical faculty members are often no more receptive to such inquiries than physicians have been to the questions they are increasingly asked by well-informed patients about proposed diagnostic and therapeutic procedures. Nonetheless, query and response are the mode of communication that precedes decisions made jointly by equals who bring different perspectives, experience, and expertise to bear upon a common problem.

Important as technical service and professional resource functions may be, the professional staff of an education unit is not likely to be content without an opportunity to engage in more than responsive activities; it also needs a chance to initiate things. In fact, on a general university campus, where most of these professionals have been trained, work undertaken as the result of individual initiative occupies most of a faculty member's time. In that setting, there is relatively little expectation that technical or even professional services will be rendered, although some regard teaching as a service that pays for the research opportunities that bring personal satisfaction as well as academic rewards. In making the move to a medical center campus, many of these nonmedical professionals have difficulty adjusting to an unfamiliar value system, one where the most prominent responsibility in the dominant clinical departments is service — to patients — and where service obligations supply research opportunities rather than diverting attention from them. Some of the transplants never recover from this cultural shock and complain endlessly about the service they must provide while missing incomparable opportunities to transform that work into descriptive research or even hypothesis testing.

But the academic function also includes responsibility for the education of students; it is, in fact, the function that distinguishes a complete faculty member from either a technician or a research worker. Although it becomes increasingly clear that health practitioners must gain greater skill as educators if they are to help their patients learn more effectively how to maintain personal health or to profit most from therapeutic interventions, very few education units have yet been invited to assist in this basic instruction of health professionals. However, most medical education units not only recognize a responsibility, but also actively seek an opportunity, to improve the pedagogic qualifications of faculty members who *are* responsible for implementing those professional programs. How to accomplish that mission is another question.

As the 1977 questionnaire revealed, there is a wide range of opinion about the work called "faculty development." The term itself is offensive to some, while others believe it may be the most important task that medical education units face. The argument is not so much whether education professionals can contribute anything to faculty understanding of educational process and skill in its application, as whether this should be accomplished through individualized work/project activities or through more formally organized programs. To become entangled in an either/or debate is fruitless, but to take no stand on the question is not very helpful either.

From time to time and place to place, educational science enthusiasts, as well as administrators frustrated by an apparent lack of faculty concern for teaching, have proposed that instruction in the art and science of pedagogy be a prerequisite to faculty appointment or a requirement before advancing to tenure rank. Although the envisioned purpose may be noble, a policy of this nature would invite disaster, not to mention a tidal wave of resistance. Furthermore, there is no reason to believe that such a requirement would be any more successful in improving teaching than obligatory participation in research projects has heightened the general level of analytic skill among medical students, or required courses in the humanities have perceptibly changed their attitudes and values.

Nonetheless, there does seem to be a place for organized and systematic programs in educational science (seminars, workshops, courses) to help faculty members who have recognized a need that can be met by such instruction, or to provoke some of the more reluctant dragons to discover that there really is something about education they can still learn. For the few who want to acquire a depth of understanding that might qualify them as educational professionals, not simply well-informed amateurs, there is also a need for advanced study opportunities that might even lead to a graduate degree. Although few of the established units have sufficient staff to mount such a full range of formal programs, the omission of any organized effort to share their expertise with health professions faculty, except through individual project work, would almost seem a neglect of professional responsibility.

A question that still keeps surfacing is whether health professions schools should independently mount faculty development programs of this kind, or should simply contract with a faculty of education to provide them. Although there is no longer any reasonable doubt that professionals from education must make a significant contribution to this effort, there is also no doubt, at least in my mind, that professional schools of education cannot do it alone or even be perceived as primary movers in the work. Faculty development of the kind most needed in health professions schools must be an integral part of the academic setting with which participants identify, not a peripheral attachment to that world; the content must be clearly related to the problems they face, not to those that require an intellectual act of transfer for perceived relevance; the language must be that of the biomedical scientist, not the "jargon" of the educational scientist. Even a graduate degree program, if it is professionally oriented, should probably be based in a health professions school or college, and not merely use that setting as a site for field work. It is not that the alternative will not work, but simply that it may not work as well, particularly if a major purpose of faculty development is to influence the educational system and not the individual participants alone.

For there are several levels at which these efforts can be aimed. The first is clearly that of *individual development,* which may attempt no more than to widen horizons, to provide new insight into the place of medical education in a university program, to stimulate an awareness of current issues in education, and to encourage familiarity with current or classic education literature that might be helpful in dealing with problems of immediate concern. At best it would go beyond a purely intellectual experience and provide the kind of emotional jolt that a Nathaniel Cantor or a Carl Rogers gave to many of us, a jolt that leads to a changed perception of the primary faculty role from one that focuses on teaching to one that is primarily concerned with learning.

At the next level are programs aimed at *instructional development,* such as curriculum organization, design of new or refinement of old teaching materials, exploitation of instructional technology, and creation of improved evaluation procedures. Along with this work on the tools of instruction there should naturally develop a concomitant conern for sharpening teacher skills in the use of the tools: analysis of classroom performance, encouragement and utilization of feedback from students and colleagues, and employment of micro-teaching exercises and comparable developmental devices.

But neither of these components will have great impact unless equal attention is given to *organizational development.* Whether they like it or not, individual teachers are part of a system. They may choose to ignore it, but only at the cost of impaired effectiveness. In fact, health professions faculty members are part of two systems, which sometimes appear to be operating asynchronously, if not actually at cross-purposes. Both Magraw with a national agenda, and Fulop with one that is worldwide, have highlighted and underscored the inescapable fact that health professions education can no longer operate in splendid isolation from the health service system of which it is part. Medical schools and medical faculty members must become better acquainted with and more responsive to the imperatives of health service needs, the organizational options that are available to meet them, and the costs as well as the benefits attending the choices that are made. A faculty development program that neglects this aspect of responsibility is at best incomplete and at worst counterproductive.

The academic system is another part of organization that needs to be seen more clearly, understood more fully, and used more effectively. Despite their preference for autonomy, both individual teachers and academic departments are part of a larger institutional organization, with checks and balances that they more often regard as abrading than as lubricating the operation. Thus a faculty development program should also aim to improve understanding of system options and limits, of constraints imposed by external forces and those generated by internal accomodation, of methods to improve interpersonal communication and the resolution of conflict, and of ways to optimize the management of resources (space, equipment, personnel, money) and minimize waste.

Even though all of these components may sound reasonable and logical, even desirable, fulfillment of a faculty development function by academic units of medical education will in the end be influenced most profoundly by a factor over which they have no direct control: the faculty reward system. Both the plentiful anecdotal accounts and occasional systematic studies support a conclusion that the higher education community rewards scholarly activity most highly (and for "scholarly activity" read "research and publication"), professional service next (and here the service may be rendered to professional organizations, the public at large, or, in health professions schools, to patients), and only last, if at all, the function of teaching.

This is not intended to suggest that medical faculties do not value good teaching; on the contrary, teaching appears regularly among the criteria for selection and promotion. Certainly no one who has served on a promotions committee can fail to be impressed by the fact that virtually all candidates for academic advancement are described as first-rate teachers. Yet everyone recognizes that this is a game played with a straight face, like admiration for the emperor's new clothes. It would take no more than the child's cry that "he's naked" to destroy the whole illusion, but there is reluctance to do so in the absence of criteria upon which to make a more sober judgment of teaching competence.

If the problem is ever to be solved, a useful place to begin might be by acknowledging that there is no single characterization of a "good" teacher, any more than there is one way to describe a "good" physician or a "good" drug; it must be done in terms of "good for what?" Since the only legitimate purpose of teaching is to facilitate learning, it would seem reasonable to begin the judgment there. Just as an investigator's familiarity with the field of study is a primary consideration in the judgment of research competence, so a teacher's knowledge of adult learning ought to enter into the appraisal of teaching competence (it goes without saying that any faculty member has already been judged to be qualified in subject matter, or the original appointment would never have been made). It would seem almost axiomatic that teachers who do not understand how students learn may have difficulty helping them to do so, yet this fact seems to have escaped many well-intentioned medical faculty members. Certainly any knowledgeable observer of the instruction that takes place in the classroom, ward, laboratory, or clinic must be alarmed by the frequency with which the transaction seems to impede as much as foster the kind of learning that is said to be its objective.

A second criterion regularly used to judge professional performance is the skill with which research workers or practitioners use the tools of the trade. Lectures, group discussions, examinations, and audiovisual aids are among the most prominent tools teachers use. Yet how often are these instructional practices directly observed and analyzed in terms of technical proficiency? Anyone who has systematically sampled medical school teaching would probably conclude that the frequency of educational malpractice is considerably greater than we might like to think.

Finally, faculty performance in a medical school is regularly weighed on the scale of scholarly creativity and inquiry, yet there is little to suggest that educational creativity and the systematic study of educational process, which should enter into the judgment of teaching competence, carry more than the weight of a feather. In fact many medical school teachers would adamantly maintain that these factors are weighed negatively, for energy invested in this sphere detracts from time and effort that could be given to other "more productive" things.

If this description is accurate — that the importance of teaching is only nominally acknowledged, that judgments are impressionistic at best and uninformed at worse, that few points are won by trying to teach better — then medical educationists who want to help teachers improve their pedagogic qualifications face an environment that impedes rather than supports this work. Plato noted centuries ago that "what is honored in a country will be cultivated there." If competence as an educator is to assume the importance it deserves in the repertoire of a medical school faculty member, then it must be honored far more than now.

And so, in the end, both the problems and the prospects have been captured by an ancient in a pithy phrase. Behavior is more likely to be influenced by what is emotionally valued than by what is rationally conceded. It is true in the education of medical students; it is equally true in the education of medical teachers.

The educational research and development community has probably gone about as far as it can in influencing the medical education system through purely intellectual discourse. Data are still necessary, but alone they are no longer sufficient to ensure further progress toward incorporating the science of learning into the art of teaching. The truth is that they never have been. Medical educationists may need to learn this hard lesson once more, and adapt to it rather than fight against it.

Adaptation, however, implies neither capitulation to external forces nor Machiavellian manipulation to change them. It simply suggests that talent, time, and effort need to be invested in work most likely to influence what is esteemed, in a manner that is least likely to be interpreted as self-serving. In the best sense it means that medical education units should aim to become the educational conscience of a medical school, seeking neither converts to a new way of life nor academic accolades, serving simply as the institutional gyroscope that helps a faculty to keep on course in fulfilling its educational mission. It is not an easy role to play, since few faculties relish being reminded of discrepancies between what they espouse and what they do. And it is certainly not without hazard, for there is a fine line between persistent pursuit of questions that need to be addressed, and constant nagging about issues that no one is prepared to face. The one is tolerable, even admirable; the other is ultimately intolerable — even grounds for divorce.

In moments of discouragement medical education unit directors and their associates may feel that this difficult balance requires the wisdom of a Solomon, the patience of a Job, and the serenity of a Gandhi. These attributes would undoubtedly help things along, but a more realistic target is simply an unswerving search for new answers to old educational questions and for ever better ways to fulfill the social, as well as the academic, purposes for which medical schools have been established. That spirit must be coupled with honest acknowledgment that not all old instructional practices are necessarily bad and all innovations good. But it does imply that educational research, development, and teacher training have change as their objective, not because existing practices are without merit, but because there is virtually nothing that cannot be improved.

Yet schools and individuals alike resist change in sometimes unpredictable but always well-rationalized ways. John Gardner has posed the dilemma we all face in these thoughtful words:

> I am always puzzled by people who talk as though the advocates of change [were] just inventing ways to disturb the peace in what would otherwise be a tranquil community. We are not seeking change for the sheer fun of it. We must change to meet the challenge of altered circumstances. Change will occur whether we like it or not. It will be either change in a good and healthy direction or change in a bad and regrettable direction. There is no tranquillity for us.
>
> We can choose not to accept the challenge, of course, but then we shall fall very rapidly into the ranks of the museum nations, and tourists from more vigorous lands will come from afar to marvel at our quaint ways.[6]

The education of medical teachers is one way to avoid that melancholy outcome.

NOTES

INDEX

NOTES

1. IDEAS WITHOUT ACTION

1. Ward Darley, "Research in Medical Education," *J. Med. Educ.* 39:97-98, 1964.

2. C. A. Theodor Billroth, *The Medical Sciences in German Universities,* trans. from the 1876 German edition *Lehren und Lernen der Medicinishen Wissenschaften* (New York: Macmillan, 1924).

3. Ibid., p. 246.

4. E. L. Holmes, address at the annual banquet of the Practitioners Club in Chicago, *J.A.M.A.* 18:114-115, 1892.

5. "Methods of Medical Instruction," (editorial), *J.A.M.A.* 18:83, 1892.

6. B. Holmes, "The Progress of Medical Education," *J.A.M.A.* 33:1567-1570, 1899.

7. W. B. Cannon, "The Case Method of Teaching Systematic Medicine," *Boston Med. Surg. J.* 142:31, 1900.

8. R. C. Cabot and E. A. Locke, "The Organization of a Department of Medicine," *Boston Med. Surg. J.* 153:461-463, 1905.

9. Cited in P. Sanazaro, "The Renaissance of AAMC Interest in Medical Education," *J. Med. Educ.* 39:229-231, 1964.

10. Ibid.

11. A. Flexner, *Medical Education in the United States and Canada*, Carnegie Foundation for the Advancement of Teaching, Bulletin no. 4 (New York, 1910), p. 53.

12. Ibid., pp. 55, 57.

13. Ibid., p. 56.

14. Ibid.

15. Ibid., pp. 57, 59.

16. Ibid., pp. 60-61.

17. E. P. Lyon, "The Relation of the Laboratory Courses to the Work of the Clinical Years," *J.A.M.A.* 66:631-633, 1916.

18. M. E. Haggerty, "The Improvement of Medical Instruction," *J. Assoc. Am. Med. Coll.* 4:42-58, 1929.

19. A. D. Hirschfelder, "Coordination in the Teaching of the Fundamental and Clinical Sciences," *J. Assoc. Am. Med. Coll.* 4:6-12, 1929.

20. I. S. Cutter, "The School of Medicine," in *Higher Education in America,* ed. R. A. Kent (Boston: Ginn, 1930).

21. R. H. Oppenheimer, "What Should the Teacher Keep in Mind in the Instruction of Medical Students?" *J. Assoc. Am. Med. Coll.* 9:360-365, 1934.

22. *Final Report of the Commission on Medical Education* (New York, 1932), pp. 3, 244.

23. W. D. Reid, *Teaching Methods in Medicine: The Application of the Philosophy of Contemporary Education to Medical School* (Newton, Mass., 1933 [privately printed]), p. 17.

24. W. D. Reid, "The Medical Teacher," *J. Assoc. Am. Med. Coll.* 7:22-28, 1932.

25. Book review, *J. Assoc. Am. Med. Coll.* 8:369, 1933.

26. R. S. Aitken, "The Teaching of Medicine," *Lancet* 225 (2), 1945.

27. R. D. Lawrence, "The Training of Clinical Teachers," *Br. Med. J.* 482-483 (2), 1950.

28. L. B. Slobody, "How to Improve Teaching in Medical Colleges," *J. Assoc. Am. Med. Coll.* 25:45-49, 1950.

29. R. Meyers, "Educational Science in Medical Teaching," *J. Med. Educ.* 29:17-30, 1954.

30. W. R. Niblett, "The Training of Teachers," *Br. Med. J.* 527, 1949.

31. Paul Klapper, "Medical Education as Education," *J. Assoc. Am. Med. Coll.* 25:314-318, 1950.

32. J. E. Deitrick and R. C. Berson, *Medical Schools in the United States at Mid-Century* (New York: McGraw-Hill, 1953), pp. 238, 328.

33. *The Training of a Doctor*, Report of the Medical Curriculum Committee of the British Medical Association (London, 1948), p. 68.

34. Abraham White, "Problems Relating to Teachers," chap. 5 in *Report of the First Teaching Institute of the Association of American Medical Colleges, J. Med. Educ.* 29, part II, July 1954.

35. W. Darley and E. Turner, "Leadership in Curriculum Planning," *J. Assoc. Am. Med. Coll.* 25:17, 1950.

36. W. M. Arnott, "The Aims of the Medical Curriculum," in *Proceedings of the First World Conference on Medical Education* (London: Oxford University Press, 1954), pp. 279-280.

37. L. Whitby, "The Challenge to Medical Education in the Second Half of the Twentieth Century," in *Proceedings of the First World Conference on Medical Education* (London: Oxford University Press, 1954), p. 11.

2. BUFFALO: IN THE BEGINNING . . .

1. E. W. Bridge, "Problems in Medical Education," mimeographed, University of Buffalo School of Medicine, 1951.

2. Ibid.

3. G. E. Miller, "Bedside Teaching for First Year Students," *J. Med. Educ.* 29:28, 1954.

4. Report of the Committee on Educational Survey to the Faculty of the Massachusetts Institute of Technology (Cambridge, Mass.: Technology Press, 1949).

5. E. W. Bridge, "Experiments in Medical Education 1951-52," mimeographed, University of Buffalo School of Medicine, 1952.

6. G. E. Miller, "Adventure in Pedagogy," *J.A.M.A.* 162: 1448-1450, 1956.

7. N. Cantor, *The Teaching ⇌ Learning Process* (New York: Dryden Press, 1953).

8. G. E. Miller, foreword to N. Cantor, *Dynamics of Learning* (reprinted by Agathon Press, New York, 1972).

9. R. A. Lyman, "Disaster in Pedagogy," *N. Engl. J. Med.* 257:504-507, 1957.

3. BUFFALO: THE PROJECT IN MEDICAL EDUCATION

1. J. H. Comroe, "The Achievements of the Institute," chap. 7 in *The Teaching of Physiology, Biochemistry, Pharmacology,* Report of the First Teaching Institute, Association of American Medical Colleges (Chicago, 1954), p. 104.

2. G. E. Miller and E. F. Rosinski, "A Summer Institute on Medical Teaching: Report of a Conference," *J. Med. Educ.* 34:449-495, 1959.

3. E. F. Rosinski and G. E. Miller, "Seminars on Medical Teaching: A Recapitulation," *J. Med. Educ.* 37:177-184, 1962.

4. Hilliard Jason, "A Study of Medical Teaching Practices," *J. Med. Educ.* 37: 1258-1284, 1962.

5. E. F. Rosinski and G. E. Miller, "A Study of Medical School Faculty Attitudes," *J. Med. Educ.* 37:112-123, 1962.

6. G. E. Miller, ed., *Teaching and Learning in Medical School* (Cambridge, Mass.: Harvard University Press, 1961).

7. B. P. Lipton, "Review of *Teaching and Learning in Medical School,*" *J.A.M.A.* 179:102, 1962.

4. INITIAL COLONIZATION

1. E. F. Rosinski and W. B. Blanton, "A System of Cataloging the Subject Matter of a Medical School Curriculum," *J. Med. Educ.* 37:1092-1100, 1962.

5. PARALLEL DEVELOPMENTS

1. J. T. Wearn, "The End Depends Upon the Beginning," *Medical Alumni Bulletin of Case Western Reserve University* 38, no. 2, 1974.

2. Ibid.

3. T. H. Ham, "Medical Education at Western Reserve University: A Progress Report for the Sixteen Years 1946-1962," *N. Engl. J. Med.* 267:868-874, 1962.

4. J. W. Harris, D. L. Horrigan, J. R. Ginther, and T. H. Ham, "Pilot Study in Teaching Hematology with Emphasis on Self-Education by the Students," *J. Med. Educ.* 37:719-736, 1962; J. R. Ginther, "Cooperative Research in Medical Education: An Example from Hematology," *J. Med. Educ.* 38:718-724, 1963.

5. T. H. Ham, *The Student as Colleague* (Ann Arbor, Mich.: University Microfilms, 1975).

6. J. H. Comroe, "Group Instruction in the Art and Techniques of Lecturing," *J. Med. Educ.* 29:39-41, 1954.

7. Alexander Robertson, "A Program of Continuing Education for Medical Educators," *Can. Med. Assoc. J.* 83:1367-1369, 1960.

8. Medical Teaching Committee of the Royal College of Physicians, Second Interim Report, *Lancet* II:132, 1955 (July).

9. J. R. Ellis, "Changes in Medical Education," *Lancet* I:813-818, 867-872, 1956 (June).

10. R. Ganzarain, G. Gil, and K. Grass, "Human Relations and the Teaching-Learning Process in Medical School," *J. Med. Educ.* 41:61-69, 1966.

11. A. Neghme, "Medical Education in the Americas," *J. Med. Educ.* 40:419-436, 1965.

12. G. Redd, "A Dental Faculty Analyzes Its Teaching Program," *J. Dent. Educ.* 12:79-83, 1948.

13. Commission on the Survey of Dentistry in the United States, *Survey of Dentistry,* Final Report of the Commission (Washington, D.C.: American Council on Education, 1961).

6. GROWTH AND INFILTRATION

1. Committee on Professional Education, *The Physician's Continuing Education* (New York: American Heart Association, 1961).

2. G. P. Berry, "Medical Education in Transition," *J. Med. Educ.* 28:17-42, 1953.

3. G. P. Berry, preface to *The Appraisal of Applicants to Medical School,* ed. H.H. Gee and J. T. Cowles (Evanston, Ill.: Association of American Medical Colleges, 1957).

4. P. J. Sanazaro, "The Placebo Effect in Medical Education," *J. Med. Educ.* 35:416, 1960.

5. H. S. Becker et al., *Boys in White* (Chicago: University of Chicago Press, 1961).

6. F. L. Husted and T. L. Hawkins, "Resident Orientation to Education: A Pilot Venture," *J. Med. Educ.* 38:111, 1963.

7. H. Jason, "A Study of the Teaching of Medicine and Surgery in a Canadian Medical School," *Can Med. Assoc. J.* 90:813-819, 1964.

7. MOBILIZING SUPPORT

1. C. McGuire, R. E. Hurley, D. Babbott, and J. S. Butterworth, "Auscultatory Skill: Gain and Retention After Intensive Instruction," *J. Med. Educ.* 39:120-131, 1964.

2. J. W. Williamson and C. McGuire, "Consecutive Case Conference: An Educational Evaluation," *J. Med. Educ.* 43:1068-1074, 1968.

3. G. E. Miller, J. S. Allender, and A. V. Wolf, "Differential Achievement with Programmed Text, Teaching Machine and Conventional Instruction in Physiology," *J. Med. Educ.* 40:817-824, 1965; J. S. Allender, L. S. Bernstein, and G. E. Miller, "Differential Achievement and Differential Cost in Programmed Instruction and Conventional Instruction in Internal Medicine," *J. Med. Educ.* 40:825-831, 1965.

4. J. W. Williamson, M. Alexander, and G. E. Miller, "Continuing Education and Patient Care Research," *J.A.M.A.* 201:938-942, 1967.

5. Advisory Committee on Health Education and Communications, *Education for Health,* U.S. Department of Health, Education, and Welfare, Public Health Service Publication no. 1430 (Washington, D.C.: U.S. Government Printing Office, 1966).

6. S. Abrahamson, J. S. Denson, and R. Wolf, "Effectiveness of a Simulator in Training Anesthesiology Residents," *J. Med. Educ.* 44:515-519, 1969.

7. G. E. Miller, "The Orthopaedic Training Study—Phase I: The Certification of Professional Competence," *Clin. Orthop.* 75:38-48, 1971; C. McGuire, "The Orthopaedic Training Study—Phase II: The Training Programs," *Clin. Orthop.* 75:49-60, 1971.

8. INTERNATIONAL REVERBERATIONS

1. L. A. Hulst, "The Hospital Bedside Teaching of Medicine," in *Proceedings of the First World Conference on Medical Education* (London: Oxford University Press, 1954), p. 401.

2. D. G. Anderson, in *Proceedings of the Second World Conference on Medical Education* (New York: World Medical Association, 1961), p. 611.

3. J. Ellis, "Final Address," in *Proceedings of the Third World Conference on Medical Education," Indian J. Med. Educ.* 7:389-398, 1968.

4. Report of the Expert Committee on Professional and Technical Education of Medical and Auxiliary Personnel, World Health Organization Technical Report Series no. 22 (Geneva, 1950), p. 22.

5. Second Report of the Expert Committee on Professional and Technical Education of Medical and Auxiliary Personnel, World Health Organization Technical Report Series no. 69 (Geneva, 1953), p. 19.

6. *The Training and Preparation of Teachers for Medical Schools with Special Regard to the Needs of Developing Countries,* Report of the Expert Committee on Professional and Technical Education of Medical and Auxiliary Personnel, World Health Organization Technical Report Series no. 337 (Geneva, 1966), p. 26.

7. Report of an Advisory Group on the Evaluation of the W.H.O. Programme for Education and Training, multilith (Geneva, 1967).

8. Report of a Consultation on Teacher Training for Health Personnel, World Health Organization, multilith (Geneva, 1969).

9. *Development of Education Programmes for the Health Professions,* W.H.O. Public Health Papers no 52 (Geneva, 1973); G. F. Miller and T. Fulop, eds., *Educational Strategies for the Health Professions,* W.H.O. Public Health Papers no 61 (Geneva, 1974).

10. *Training and Preparation of Teachers for Schools of Medicine and Allied Health Sciences,* Report of a W.H.O. Study Group, Technical Report Series no. 521 (Geneva, 1973).

9. ASSIMILATION AND INTEGRATION

1. J. F. Steiger, Report on a One Year Fellowship Program at Different Institutions of Research in Medical Education in North America 1971/1972, Institute of Research in Medical Education and Evaluation, University of Bern, 1972.

2. P. G. Bashook, Memorandum from AERA/SIG/HPE Chairperson to Members, July 21, 1976.

3. Committee on Goals and Priorities Final Report, *Evaluation in the Continuum of Medical Education,* National Board of Medical Examiners (Philadelphia, 1973).

4. P. J. Sanazaro, "Research in Patient Care: Its Relevance to Medical Education" (editorial), *J. Med. Educ.* 39:1121-1122, 1964.

5. H. Jason, H. B. Slotnick, and R. D. Lefever, Faculty Development Survey Final Report, Association of American Medical Colleges (Washington, D.C. 1977).

6. W. Darley and A. S. Cain, "A Proposal for a National Academy of Continuing Medical Education," *J. Med. Educ.* 36:33-37, 1961.

7. B. V. Dryer, "Lifetime Learning for Physicians," *J. Med. Educ.,* Suppl. 37, June 1962.

8. P. B. Storey, J. W. Williamson, and C. H. Castle, *Continuing Medical Education: A New Emphasis* (Chicago: American Medical Association, 1968).

9. P. J. Sanazaro, "An Agenda for Research in Medical Education," *J.A.M.A.* 197:979-984, 1966.

10. J. Bryant, *Health and the Developing World* (Ithaca, N.Y.: Cornell University Press, 1969).

10. PROBLEMS AND PROSPECTS

1. J. Steiner, "Educational Research for Decision-Making," Proceedings of the Fourth Pan American Conference on Medical Education, multilith (University of Toronto, 1973), p. 23.

2. G. E. Miller, "A Perspective on Research in Medical Education," *J. Med. Educ.* 45:694-699, 1970.

3. Steiner, "Educational Research," p. 23.

4. E. D. Pellegrino, "Research in Medical Education: The Views of a Friendly Philistine," *J. Med. Educ.* 46:750-756, 1971.

5. R. M. Magraw, D. M. Fox, and J. L. Weston, "Health Professions Education and Public Policy: A Research Agenda," *J. Med. Educ.* 53:539-546, 1978.

6. John. W. Gardner, *No Easy Victories* (New York: Harper & Row, 1968), p. 50.

INDEX

Aagaard, George, 120
AAMC, *see* Association of American Medical Colleges
Abrahamson, Stephen, 35-36, 82, 120, 126, 143, 191; and Educational Research Center (Buffalo), 45, 49, 50; at Stanford University, 86-91, 131; at University of Southern California, 129, 142, 184, 185
Adams, William R., 102
Administration: of medical education units, 177-178, 180, 183-188, 206
Africa, 160, 163, 167
Albany Medical College, 114, 128, 146
Aldrich, Malcolm, 43
Alway, Robert, 87
American Academy of Microbiology, 114
American Association of Dental Schools, 111-112
American College of Physicians, 200
American College of Radiology, 114
American Educational Research Association (AERA), 189-190, 212
American Heart Association (AHA), 115, 136-138, 145
American Medical Association (AMA), 198-200
Anderson, Alexander, 137
Anderson, Donald, 53, 127, 152
Anderson, Lester, 36, 45
Andrew, Barbara, 191
Anesthesiologists: training of, 143
Arnott, W. Melville, 20
Assessment, *see* Evaluation
Association of American Medical Colleges (AAMC), 8, 116-127, 152, 192-199; committees of, 8-9, 12, 18, 119; Teaching Institutes, 62, 117-118, 121; divisions of, 121, 123, 192, 194-197; Conference on Research in Medical Education, 188-189; Groups of, 195
Association for the Study of Medical Education (ASME), 107
Association of Hospital Directors of Medical Education, 114
Audiovisual aids, *see* Technology, educational
Australia, 163, 171, 201
Autonomous Metropolitan University of Mexico City, 201
Autonomy, departmental, 209-211, 219

Baltimore City Medical Society, 114
Barrows, Howard, 130, 142
Becker, Donald, 48, 78, 79
Ben Gurion University, 201
Bennett, Granville, 92, 94
Berry, George Packer, 117-118
Billroth, Theodor, 5-6
Biomedical research, *see* Research, biomedical
Blair, Murray, 48, 78
Bloom, Benjamin, 29, 96, 102, 127
Boston University, 15-16
Bowers, John Z., 198
Boylan, John, 33
Bridge, Edward, 21-23, 25, 27-29, 45, 78, 109
British Life Assurance Trust Center for Health and Medical Education, 170
Brody, Harold, 47
Brown, Clement, 137
Bruner, Jerome, 102
Bryant, John, 202
Budgets, *see* Educational research, funds for; Funds
Bunnell, Ivan, 45
Bureau of State Services, 140-141, 144, 145
Butrov, V. N., 156

Cabot, Richard C., 7
California Medical Association, 114
Canada, 47, 67, 105, 114, 201

231